FROM COAST TO COAST, EVERYONE IS TALKING ABOUT

THE INCREDIBLE STARCH-BLOCKER DIET.

Dr. John Marshall, author of THE ORIGINAL STARCH-BLOCKER DIET, is the world-famous biochemist and authority on starch chemistry and enzymology who discovered the starch-blocker ten years ago and who has since developed this revolutionary breakthrough permanent weight-loss plan—published here for the first time.

The effect of the starch-blocker is simple and limited. It nutritionally inhibits the action of alpha amylase, the digestive enzyme that changes starch into glucose (blood sugar), which is then used by the body as calories Changing starch into calories is the only function of this enzyme. When the enzyme is stopped from "doing the job," the starch you eat is not converted into calories, and ultimately into fat.

Therefore: if you eat a bowl of spaghetti with tomato sauce, you absorb the calories only from the sauce—not the spaghetti. If you have an English muffin with butter, only the calories from the butter count.

·THE ORIGINAL·
STARCH-BLOCKER DIET

For the very first time—
eat without absorbing calories

by Dr. John Marshall

with Robert Lemon

A JOAN HITZIG MCDONELL BOOK

Published by
Dell Publishing Co., Inc.
1 Dag Hammarskjold Plaza
New York, New York 10017

This book is not intended as a prescription or as a substitute for the advice of a physician. Persons who may require medical care should consult a physician before attempting a special dietary plan.

Dell ® TM 681510, Dell Publishing Co., Inc.

ISBN: 0-440-04078-7

Printed in the United States of America

First printing—July 1982

Table of Contents

PART ONE—
THE DIET YOU'LL LOVE
1—The New World Of Weight Loss 15
2—How The Starch-Blocker Works 33

PART TWO—
DISCOVERY, DEVELOPMENT, TESTING
3—Discovery 47
4—Development Of The Starch-Blocker 55
5—How We Know The Starch-Blocker Works ... 65

PART THREE—
HOW THE STARCH-BLOCKER CAN HELP YOU
6—How To Use The Starch-Blocker 81
7—How Not To Use The Starch-Blocker 115
8—The Starch-Blocker Diet 121
9—How To Begin Your Program 225

PART FOUR—
WHY YOU DIDN'T LOSE WEIGHT BEFORE AND WHY YOU SHOULD NOW
10—What's Wrong With Other Diets 241
11—Why It's Important To Lose Weight 253

PART FIVE—
ANSWERS AND INTERVIEWS
12—Answers To Your Questions 263
13—Interviews With Starch-Blocker Users 273

About The Authors

J. John Marshall, PhD

J. John Marshall was born in Edinburgh, Scotland. After earning a BSC in chemistry from the University of Edinburgh and a PhD in biochemistry from Heriot-Watt University, Edinburgh, he moved to the United States. In 1969 he began work as a Research Associate at the University of Miami. In 1973 he was appointed Director of Biochemical Research at Howard Hughes Medical Institute in Miami, Florida. He held this position until 1980. During that period he also served as Associate Professor of Biochemistry and Assistant Professor of Medicine at University of Miami Medical School. At the present time he is a faculty member of the Department of Microbiology at the University of Notre Dame.

Dr. Marshall has conducted research in all areas of starch chemistry, bio-chemistry and enzymology and is considered one of the world's authorities on these subjects. His bibliography lists over 100 publications, numerous U.S. patents and several books, including major works such as *Studies on the Enzymic Degradation of Polysaccharides; Studies on Carbohydrate Metabolizing Enzymes: The Beta-Glucanase System of Malted Barley; Action of Amylolytic Enzymes on a Chromogenic Substrate; A New Approach to the Use of Enzymes in Starch Technology; An Introduction to Protein Purification; Naturally Occurring Inhibitors of a-Amylase; Purification and Properties of Phaseolamin, an Inhibitor of a-Amylase from the Kidney Bean, Phaseolus vulgaris; Assay of a-Amylase Inhibitor Ac-*

Preface

This book is the complete account of a great dietary breakthrough which has come to be known as the Starch-Blocker™ Special Legume Protein Concentrate.

The Starch-Blocker concept was refined and made a practical reality by the world famous biochemist, J. John Marshall, Ph.D. The concept took twelve years to research and develop. Since its introduction the Starch-Blocker innovation has been in use by tens of thousands of people. The product is thoroughly described in this book. Results have been reported as being excellent to spectacular. Comments such as "It's so simple and easy it's almost like not being on a diet" have been common.

The dramatic and widespread acceptance of Dr. Marshall's dietary innovation has attracted a great amount of interest from the public, the medical profession and manufacturers as well. Of paramount importance in any dietary regime is the genuineness and quality of the product being applied. This should be kept in mind when a brand of product is finally selected for use in a diet.

This book reports on important scientific facts and the personal experiences of many dedicated people. It is recommended that you read this book twice—one time to capture the central theme, and one time to thoroughly understand and be able to apply the concepts and important facts that have made Dr. Marshall's dietary breakthrough a practical reality.

Introduction

By Guy Colpron, M.D.

Fat. Obese. Overweight. Regardless of the thousands of excuses that come and go, a fact of life remains: The basic cause of being overweight is the intake of calories beyond the needs of the body. Eating proper foods in the right amounts and lesser amounts of bad foods is the only valid approach to weight control. It's a fact of life. It may sound simple but we know it isn't. And today's lifestyle complicates the situation. Rich foods, "empty" calorie snacks and the lack of quality exercise are a few of the culprits that have put extra pounds of fat on millions of people. It is estimated that at least 35% of adults in the United States are overweight. This figure increases after age forty.

As a population, we're very sensitive about our overweight condition. This is borne out by the number of fad diets which have appeared in recent years. Many of these diets have been "overnight" successes only because of the fast results they offered, however temporary they are. At best, many of these diets may produce rapid loss of body water. The long term use of many of these diets may result in nutritional as well as body fluid imbalances. They can also lead to extreme anxiety when the diet becomes more of a battle than a rewarding experience.

For several important reasons, Dr. Marshall's development represents a refreshing and rational approach to weight control.

First, it is a natural protein that is commonly found

in kidney beans, other legumes and cereal grains. Therefore, it offers a natural alternative to drugs which have been widely used in the past.

There are other good reasons that favor and support Dr. Marshall's innovation. For example, the Starch-Blocker special legume protein concentrate works naturally to aid only in the nutritional inhibition of starch digestion. It does not interfere with the digestion of other nutrients. Now a person's dietary regime can include an abundant array of starch-containing foods which previously had to be avoided. A meal can be diverse and satisfying as well as nutritious.

Since using this remarkable new substance, it has been possible for many patients to stick with their programs. One patient, for example, was able to lose in excess of 100 pounds on this program, but was unsuccessful on previous attempts. He even stated that he didn't feel that he was actually on a diet. Also my patients are now able to maintain their new lower weight level because they can now use the Starch-Blocker product for long term support.

Finally, Dr. Marshall's innovative approach is easy to follow. One tablet before a meal containing starch is the basic requirement. How simple! Of course, as with all things moderation is the rule—to apply here as well. But the fact is that countless thousands of overweight people now have available to them a natural dietary aid that makes ongoing, long term weight control a reality.

PART ONE

The Diet You'll Love

CHAPTER ONE

The New World Of Weight Loss

I have never been on a diet before," the nervous college student blurts to the placid older woman as they wait in the springtime Indiana sun for the weight-loss clinic to open its doors. "Being on a diet isn't too bad. *Is* it?" she implores. "I mean, in some ways, it's really pretty *easy*. *Isn't* it?"

"Not in any way I know of, honey," says the older woman.

"Well, I don't mean 'easy,' actually," the younger woman allows. "What I mean is, it's not really what you'd call 'awful,' is it?"

The older woman, a sparkling expanse of color in her sun-illumined Hawaiian muu-muu, ponders the question at some length, then answers accurately, if not entirely charitably.

"Yes, I'd say 'awful' is a pretty good word for it." The student groans, her fears confirmed, prompting the older woman to be rather more encouraging. "Well," she says, "maybe all it is, is . . . 'dreadful'—you know, like a bad cold." The student's lips begin to tremble. "But not dreadful all the time," quickly amends the older woman. "Sometimes it's just . . ." she gropes for a kinder adjective ". . . maybe a *little bit* dreadful."

"I'm hungry," moans the student, as she slumps against the side of the building.

"Now don't get down in the dumps, honey." The older woman, a 46-year-old hospital housekeeper, pats the student's shoulder. "Maybe this diet will be different from the others. I heard from a girl in my exercise class that they've got a new kind of pill at this clinic that lets you eat more."

The 22-year-old student, whose midsection had begun to balloon from too many cheese Danish study breaks when she began classes at an Indiana community college, perks up. "Then maybe this particular diet *won't* be so bad?"

"It can't be worse than the stuff I used to try. Why, in the old days, it was just about impossible to lose weight with all the gimmicks they used. In the early 1960s, they had us drinking those diet milkshakes that were just sugar and milk and vitamins. You drank those and skipped meals—but the milkshakes had more calories than a steak and french fries. Then I got into those diet candies that were supposed to kill your appetite. They killed it for food and made you hungry for candy. Then my doctor put me on diet pills. They're great, if you like being a nervous wreck. I went on an all-banana diet, an all-meat diet, then a bunch of diets named after rich suburbs. I tried counting calories and counting carbohydrates. I ate fiber and drank protein and sucked little fructose candies.

"Here's how all those diets work. One—you pay somebody to go on their diet. Two—you lose weight. Three—you get hungry and go off the diet. Four—you gain more weight than ever. Five—you pay somebody *else* to go on *his* diet."

The student, product of a suspicious era, cries, "It's a conspiracy!"

"No, honey. It's just people. They like to eat."

The older woman has liked food—how it looks, how it tastes, how it feels, how it fills—for as long as she can remember. For the first 33 years of her life, she was able to eat as much of it as she wanted, and still was able to maintain a normal weight. At 5′6″, she was never far from 130 pounds. She was happy with her appearance and with her role in life as a housekeeper on a maternity ward and the mother of nine children. After the birth of her last baby, though, in 1962, she felt exhausted, and her weight began to soar. She graduated from chunky to chubby to bulbous to obese in just over a year. For several months, her doctor prescribed a thyroid preparation, which seemed to help. Because of medical complications, however, she had to stop taking it. Then her appetite became overpowering and she began overeating. She developed problems with low blood sugar, and felt tired most of the time. As the food was piled in, the weight piled on. Even when she restricted her diet, however, and ate a mere 1,000 calories per day, or about half of the amount generally eaten by the average woman, she continued to gain weight. Gaining while going hungry discouraged her, prompting her to be careless about her eating habits.

By the early 1970s she had reached a plateau of 232 pounds. And 232 pounds, give or take the weight of her muu-muu, is what she weighs on this day, as she stands with a 157-pound student outside the weight-loss clinic.

When the doors open, the two women enter the building, and enter into a new way of life. This late spring day in 1981 can be called, with absolutely no exaggeration, historic. It is a historic day not just for these two women, but for millions of overweight people.

The Starch-Blocker Is A First!

The two women have become a part of history by being among the first people to use a remarkable, newly-recognized nutritional substance: the "starch-blocker."

The two women have entered into a program that uses a natural protein which nutritionally inhibits the absorption of starch calories. Never before, in the entire history of mankind's scientific exploration of diet and nutrition, has any substance been found that keeps calorie-laden food that is eaten from being converted into energy and fat. *The starch-blocker is a "first."*

Because of this discovery, these two women, and all the other people in the world, will now be able to eat starchy foods, such as bread or potatoes or spaghetti or cereal, and not gain weight from the starch contained in them.

This starch-blocking protein, discovered in the

1930s, was finally developed in the 1970s, after years of study and research, as a dietary aid. The substance can now make weight control possible for millions of overweight people. The heretofore almost hopeless "battle of the bulge" may soon end in victory for millions, perhaps billions, of people.

Virtually all weight loss diets prior to the discovery of the starch-blocker were based around eating a small number of calories, which is very difficult for most people to do for any extended length of time. No amount of diet-cola, or fiber, or liquefied protein, or fructose candies will satisfy the natural urges of the average dieter for long periods of time. If these approaches really worked, untold millions of people would not still be overweight.

In fact, no weight loss diet previously devised has proven to be the final solution to obesity. Because of this, a new fad diet has emerged literally every year. Year in and year out, people try new diets, lose a little weight, then soon regain it because of the difficulty of staying on the diet.

The starch-blocker weight control program, however, is different from all the denial-oriented diets. It is different because of the simple fact that it employs a substance—the starch-blocker—that allows the dieter to eat foods that do not become calories. One tablet of the starch-blocker, taken with a meal, will nutritionally inhibit most all the starch calories contained in that meal. For example, a person using the starch-blocker can eat a meal composed of normal helpings of roast turkey, dressing with gravy, a baked potato, a dinner salad, a hot roll, green beans, and tapioca pudding, *and still lose weight,* because most all of the starchy calories in this starchy meal *will be eliminated!*

The starch-blocker is used most effectively in conjuction with a prudent, moderate diet, one that the dieter should never abandon. There is no need to use the substance as part of a temporary "crash" diet. "Crash" diets have been popular because, until now, almost all dieting has been based on deprivation, hunger, and culinary monotony, and has therefore been a painful experience that most people want to end as quickly as possible. But "crash" diets of any variety are unhealthy, unhappy, generally unsuccessful undertakings, and are not endeavors that the starch-blocker should be a part of. The quick weight loss diet we recommend reaches a maximum of about 1,200 calories, 700 of which are starch calories that are nutritionally inhibited.

The starch-blocker could be used, of course, to eliminate almost *all* calories from the diet—if the dieter ate almost 100 percent starch. But this would be a ridiculous thing to do. *It should never be forgotten that a proper diet must not only keep one at a desired weight, but must also provide all the nutrients needed to insure optimum health and well-being.*

Why Millions of People Need the Starch-Blocker

Food, besides providing vitamins and minerals, consists of three basic categories: (1) proteins, which provide energy, and also provide the body's cells with "building materials"; (2) fats, which help digestion, provide slowly-used energy and essential nutrients; and

(3) carbohydrates, which provide energy that is quickly used, or stored in the liver and muscles—or stored as fat. Digestible carbohydrates are made up of two categories: sugars and starches.

The starch-blocker affects the digestion of only one of these categories of food—that category, of course, is starch. Starch is found in a great many foods, but is in greatest abundance in grain foods, such as breads and pasta and cereal and rice, and vegetables, including potatoes and corn and beans, and in many fruits. There are vitamins and minerals present in starchy foods, but these nutrients are *not a part of the starch itself*. Starch alone is strictly a fuel for energy. It basically provides "*empty calories.*" If more starch is eaten than is used for energy, it can become fat.

Most people, unfortunately, eat more of this starchy fuel than they need for energy, which is one reason that so many people are overweight.

The average person eats about half of his or her caloric intake as carbohydrates, and the rest as protein and fat. Of the carbohydrates that people eat, about half comes from sugars, and half comes from starch. People generally eat about one-fourth of their diets, then, as starch.

Expressed in terms of weight, or as grams, people eat about 250 to 350 grams of carbohydrates per day. About half of these carbohydrates, as we said, are starch. Expressed in terms of calories, this amounts to about 1,000 to 1,400 calories per day from carbohydrates, with about 500 to 700 calories per day coming from starch.

This is more carbohydrate intake, and therefore more starch intake, than most people need. The federal government recommends that people eat only about 100 grams of carbohydrates per day, which amounts to about 400 calories of carbohydrates. The average person, then, is eating two to three times as many carbohydrates as he or she needs. And many people eat even more than this.

The starch-blocker can help to reduce the caloric overload from this over-consumption of starch. By taking the starch-blocker with one's meals, the average person would eliminate about one-fourth of his or her caloric intake. *This very substantial reduction of calories should enable people to maintain a desired weight!* No special dieting, and certainly no crash dieting, should be needed. Taking the starch-blocker with meals is equivalent to cutting one's caloric intake *by about one-fourth!*

If a person eats a moderate or low amount of starch, but eats too many total calories because of eating too much protein, fat or sugar, the starch-blocker will lower the total calories digested by reducing the number of calories derived from starch. Therefore, almost anyone who is overweight, even people whose "excess baggage" does not come from overeating of *starch*, can benefit by blocking starch calories.

People who are only slightly overweight should be able to take off their extra four or five pounds with only occasional use of the starch-blocker.

Using the starch-blocker can be of special benefit to people who are significantly overweight. These people seem more prone than near-normal-weight people to eating too many carbohydrates. Many overeaters seem to crave the textures, tastes and "filling ability" of breads, noodles and starchy vegetables. Many physicians and nutritionists, including almost all who recommend very high-protein diets, theorize that people who tend toward overweight crave carbohydrates because they have metabolic imbalances. These doctors believe that many overweight people secrete too much insulin, the hormone that helps regulate blood-sugar levels, when they eat carbohydrates. This extra insulin is thought to make these people even more hungry, and to aid the conversion of blood sugar to fat.

Dr. Carlton Fredericks is one of the many nutritionists who believes that many people do not digest carbohydrates properly. Dr. Fredericks believes that many overweight people are prone to "over-efficient conversion of starch and sugar into fat."

Dr. Fredericks and many other health professionals urge overweight people to significantly limit their intake of starch and sugar. No doctor, however, has ever been able to recommend any way to achieve this limiting of carbohydrates—other than to recommend self-denial of the foods that many overweight people love. The starch-blocker, of course, is the tool that these people can use to reduce their caloric absorption *without sacrificing their enjoyment* of much-appreciated foods.

How the Starch-Blocker Works

The starch-blocker that we have developed is an extract of raw kidney beans, a naturally-derived protein that is as safe as it is effective.

There is also starch-blocking protein in other plants, particularly in other raw beans, but this special protein is most abundant in the kidney bean. The starch-blocker is an organic product, one not synthesized from various chemicals in a laboratory. Because it is merely a part of the kidney bean, the starch-blocker is a food product.

The protein in kidney beans that blocks starch digestion has, of course, always been there. If kidney beans are cooked, as they virtually always are when prepared for people to eat, most of the starch-blocking protein is destroyed. That, of course, is why you can not eat a tub of three-bean salad every day and still look like Twiggy.

We strongly advise people not to eat raw kidney beans, because there are other substances in raw kidney beans that can be harmful. These harmful substances are deactivated by heat during cooking. To be safe and effective, the starch-blocker must be derived from kidney beans through a complex laboratory procedure.

The starch-blocker works by interfering with the starch-digesting function of a digestive enzyme. Enzymes are substances that stimulate chemical changes in other substances. Digestive enzymes are found most commonly in the body's digestive juices, and generally are produced by the pancreas.

The enzyme which digests starch is called alpha amylase (pronounced: al′-fuh am′-uh-lace). This enzyme is found in the digestive tract. The greatest concentration of the enzyme is in the first part of the small intestine, the duodenum. Therefore, the vast majority of starch digestion takes place in the duodenum.

The starch-blocker combines with this enzyme called

alpha amylase, leaving it inactive, and unable to break down starch.

If the starch-blocker were *not* present in the intestine, the alpha amylase would combine with the *starch*, rather than the starch-blocker, and digest it. This digested starch would then be absorbed, and either used as energy, or stored in the liver or muscles, *or stored as fat.*

When the starch-blocker *is present,* though, the starch that is eaten simply passes through the digestive tract and is excreted.

There are no known harmful effects from the starch-blocker. Because this starch-blocking protein is a natural substance that is found in many foods, its actions are completely compatible with the body's normal functions.

The starch-blocker is confined to the digestive tract, and does not travel anywhere else in the body. It does not enter the bloodstream.

The starch-blocker does not inhibit the absorption of nonstarch nutrients from foods. The vitamins and minerals and proteins in a potato, for example, are digested in a completely normal manner, since they are digested and converted by enzymes other than the starch-digesting enzyme, alpha-amylase. This *lack of effect* by the starch-blocker on food substances other than starch is, of course, why we so strongly urge consumption of a nutritious, moderate diet with the use of the starch-blocker—the starch-blocker is not a magic potion that will miraculously transform sugary, fatty and chemicalized junk foods into nourishing "manna from heaven." The starch-blocker will stop the conversion of starch into calories. And that is absolutely all it will do.

For most people, though, this action is enough.

Like most other important discoveries, the starch-blocker took years to develop. During that time, many tests and experiments were done to determine effectiveness, safety and the feasbility of commercial production.

We first began working with the starch-blocker in 1971.

During the eleven years we worked on the substance, we continually found better ways to extract a purer, more active formulation. We conducted many animal experiments and worked with physicians conducting human studies of the product, in order to be positive that the starch-blocker was as effective as it possibly could be, and to become absolutely certain that use of it would cause no negative effects.

Our highest hopes for the substance were realized in test after test.

Animal Experiments

One of the first experiments we conducted was to administer the starch-blocker to growing laboratory animals, fed a normal diet of Purina Laboratory Chow, to see if it would retard their weight gain. It did, *by about 11 percent,* compared to a "control" group of animals. (A "control" group, for those not familiar with the term, is a group in any experiment that does not receive the substance being tested. At the end of the experiment, the condition of the group that was tested is compared to that of the "control" group.)

Our next important experiment involved administering the starch-blocker to growing animals who were fed a relatively high-starch diet. This time, the animals gained about *20 percent less weight* than a control group of growing animals.

Finally, we did an experiment with full-grown animals that had just come off a weight-loss diet, one that had caused them to lose weight. Some of the animals that had just come off the diet were given a normal diet, some were given a high starch diet, some were given a normal diet with the starch-blocker, and some were given a high-starch diet with the starch-blocker. The animals given a normal diet *without* the starch-blocker and those given a high-starch diet *without* the starch-blocker regained more weight than they had lost during the previous weight loss diet. Those given a normal diet *with the starch-blocker* regained only 91 percent of their original body weight, and those given a starchy diet with the starch-blocker regained only 89 percent of their original body weight!

We tried similar experiments with other animals, and achieved even better results. No side effects ever occurred during any of the experiments, and a nine-month "chronic toxicity" study revealed that no organ or tissue damage of any kind had taken place that we were able to determine during the experiments. In all of the thousands of administrations of the substance that were performed over the years on animals, no negative effects from it ever were recorded, confirming our assumption that the starch-blocker, an organic product that doesn't enter the bloodstream, is a totally safe substance, with effects that are limited to the blocking of starch calories.

When we were certain that we had developed a totally safe and very active product, we collaborated with physicians on human studies of the starch-blocker. These clinical studies were as gratifying as the animal experiments had been.

The physicians conducting the clinical studies found that dieters who used the starch-blocker could *eat more calories* than a group of control dieters, but were able to *lose more weight* than those people. This, of course, was what we were expecting, but it still was pleasing to see the laborious development of the product finally become an exciting, practical factor in people's lives. Many of the people who took part in the studies had previously tried very hard on their diets, but had simply not been able to maintain a normal weight. Many were very discouraged from their attempts to lose weight. Some of these people had serious health problems that were associated with their chronic obesity.

We found that patients could eat up to 1,200 calories per day, if the starch-blocker were taken with meals, and still lose weight at a very rapid rate. The amount of weight loss varied from person to person, of course, depending upon the person's weight, degree of physical activity, rate of metabolism, and consistency in adhering to the diet. The majority of the patients, though, lost between one-half and three-fourths of one pound per day during a seven-week testing period. Some of the patients lost weight relatively slowly, but one patient, to our surprise, lost 18¼ pounds in one week! This patient, because of the abnormally high weight loss, was excluded from the scoring of the test results. The full test results are described in detail in a following chapter.

Even more pleasing to us than the amount of weight that was lost by the people during the test, though, was the relative ease with which it was lost. Most of these people had suffered during the loss of every pound on all of the other diets they had tried. The creators of these diets had, of course, promised these people, in books and articles and on television, that "at last a painless, no-hunger solution" to dieting had been discovered. But these discouraged, overweight people had found out, time after time, that all of these "painless" diets were based on *self-denial.* They had found out there is *nothing* painless about denial.

The relative ease of the starch-blocker weight loss program is extremely encouraging to us. It is quite apparent—at least to anyone other than a diet-guru who is peddling a spurious "no-hunger" plan—that it is the *difficulty* of most diets that makes them unsuccessful. Most of us can be thin by always eating with a great deal of prudence. But, face facts: Who's always prudent? Who's always perfect? Not many of us, of course, are. And people with a tendency to be overweight are especially prone to dietary imperfection.

One can, as have diet-gurus over the decades, insist that dieters rearrange their emotional or metabolic makeup. There is, however, only one catch to insisting that people alter their emotional or physical characteristics: It rarely works.

In the human studies of the starch-blocker, we found that people were able to achieve very significant weight losses, week after week, because they are able to satisfy their urges to eat. When they became hungry, they simply ate a starchy meal and took a starch-blocker tablet. They didn't have as much of a problem with hunger as do most dieters, because their stomachs tended to be much more full.

Two of the people in the study who mastered the starch-blocking weight loss technique very well were a young college student, whose weight problem was new to her, and a 46-year-old woman—whose overweight condition was not new to her at all.

Lucky?

It is a mid-June morning, cloudy but warm, as the two women, the college student and the older woman, await their regular weight clinic meeting. Both of them, five weeks after beginning the starch-blocker weight loss program, are noticeably thinner.

"I've lost 13 pounds" says the student, "but she's lost about 24." The student smiles at the older woman, who now wears a belt with her muu-muu.

"We're just getting started," says the older woman. "You come back again in a couple of months and I'll look like I used to."

The student, who had seemed so apprehensive only a few weeks before, now looks as if she feels in control of the condition of her body, and of her own ability to regulate her eating habits.

"If I'd have known it would be this easy," she says, "I would have done this a year ago."

"Honey," says the older woman, who had tried to lose weight so hard, for so long, "they didn't have any starch-blocker a year ago.

"You're just lucky," she says to the student with a smile, "and you know it."

"Luck has nothing to do with it," protests the student. "I'm a careful dieter!"

"Not lucky? Tell me what you ate yesterday."

The student pulls her diet diary from her purse and reads from it. "Breakfast: a poached egg, fried potatoes, a waffle with low-calorie syrup, and a starch-blocker. Lunch: a turkey sandwich, navy bean soup, rice pilaf, low-calorie bread pudding, and a starch-blocker. Dinner: filet of sole, macaroni with a light cheese sauce, a baked potato, a salad, and a starch-blocker. For snacks, I had English muffins, cinnamon toast, and vegetable sticks."

"Like I said," says the older woman. *"You're lucky!"* They both laugh, as the doors to the weight loss clinic swing open.

CHAPTER TWO

How The Starch-Blocker Works

The way the starch-blocker works is really very simple. The starch-blocker works with commonly understood principles of digestion and nutrition.

How Your Body Receives Energy

All physical activity in the universe involves the same basic transaction—energy is exchanged from one source to another. Energy enters our systems from many sources. It comes from the sun, from food and water, and from the air. Our bodies are able to transform these energy-giving entities into the vitality that sustains life. This energy exchange with the environment is known as "metabolism."

Food is our primary source of energy. Energy from the sun and air and water and earth are "stored" in food in the form of chemicals. Our bodies are able to change this stored energy into physical activity. This metabolic transformation of energy is accomplished by a series of biochemical transactions. These biochemical transactions begin with the process known as digestion.

We digest most of the food that we eat, transferring its chemicals into our cells, which then use those chemicals to perform physical actions, such as, for example, muscular contractions, or the production of heat. Often the chemicals in foods that we eat are changed into other types of chemicals during this digestive process. Some of the food that we eat remains undigested, or unused by the body, because it is an indigestible foodstuff, such as cellulose (fiber), or because the body lacks the chemicals needed to break down the food.

Digestion, of course, is performed by the digestive system, a series of organs centered around the gastrointestinal tract, the approximately 25-foot-long "hollow tube" through which food passes. The digestive system consists of the mouth, esophagus, stomach, small intestine, large intestine, rectum, and anus, through which food travels. The digestive system also involves organs such as the pancreas, salivary glands, gall bladder and liver, which contribute digestive fluids to the gastrointestinal tract.

If a person eats more food than the body needs for energy, this additional food energy is stored by the body. Some of this energy is stored in the liver and muscles as "glycogen," a substance which supplies short-term energy reserve. Long-term energy reserve is stored as fatty tissue. This fatty tissue is, of course, what we identify as "extra weight."

The using of this stored fatty tissue is what makes us take off weight. The key to successful weight-loss dieting, then, is simply to cause the body to "burn" its own stored energy. This can be done by requiring normal demands for energy from the body, while denying the body the amount of food needed to meet these energy demands—this will force the body to "burn" its own stored fat for energy. The burning of this stored fat will provide energy in an easily usable form.

Before the discovery of the starch-blocker, the only way to accomplish the burning of body fat was to deprive oneself of foods, because there was no known way to prevent the body from converting consumed food energy—otherwise known as "calories"—into either body energy or *body fat*. Now, however, we can intervene in the digestive process in a unique, unprecedented way. We can nutritionally inhibit *the digestion of starch calories.*

Does the Body Need Starch?

Often, people who are not particularly familiar with nutritional science express their concern that depriving the body of starch is depriving it of a necessary, important substance. Nothing could be further from the truth. The body does not need starch. It needs the energy that is stored in all foods, including starchy foods, but this energy comes in several forms other than starch.

Specifically, food energy comes in the form of fats, proteins and carbohydrates (carbohydrates consist of sugars and starch). Each of these food components has special characteristics, but each can be digested by the body to provide physical energy.

Fats are substances found in plant and animal foods

that consist of glycerol molecules linked to three molecules of fatty acids. Fats also include oils, which are fats that melt at room temperature. A small amount of fats in the diet is necessary. Most doctors and nutritionists agree that the average person's consumption of fat is too high. The average person eats almost half of his or her dietary calories as fat, which most health professionals believe is an excessive amount. This excess fat is believed to contribute to cardiovascular diseases. Other doctors believe it also contributes to certain forms of cancer. A more prudent percentage of fat-calories in the diet is generally considered to be about 25 percent, or less.

Proteins are composed of chains of chemical building units called "amino acids." There are generally believed to be 22 types of amino acids, and the body requires all 22 types in order to be able to build and repair its tissues. Proteins are unique in their ability to provide these "building blocks." The body can manufacture many of the amino acids, but we are dependent upon food to provide eight of these amino acids. Proteins are present in many foodstuffs, and are found in a high quantity in certain grains and vegetables, and in an especially high quantity in animal products, such as meat, fish and milk. Proteins not only provide the cells with "building materials," but also with nutrients that are used to supply energy, making proteins an especially desirable food component.

The third major form of foodstuff, carbohydrates, which consist of sugars and starch, is the food that can be most easily transformed by the body into energy, because it is the food that is most easily digested.

Carbohydrates consist of three categories, depending

upon the degree of complexity of their molecules. The categories are: (1) monosaccharides, (2) disaccharides, and (3) polysaccharides. "Mono-," as you may know, means "one," "di-" means "two," and "poly-" means "many". A monosaccharide, then, is a carbohydrate made up of one glucose molecule, and a disaccharide is made of two glucose molecules, and a polysaccharide is made up of more than two glucose molecules. These categories are also often described as "simple" or "complex." Monosaccharides and disaccharides are "simple" carbohydrates, while polysaccharides are "complex" carbohydrates. Starches, as you might have guessed, are very complex carbohydrates. Sugars come from many sources, including fruits and milk and grains. Different foods contain various amounts and types of sugars. For example, fructose, or sugar from fruit, is one of the simple carbohydrates. Other examples of simple sugars are glucose and galactose. Some examples of disaccharides are sucrose, or cane sugar; lactose, or milk sugar; and maltose, or malted grain cereal sugar.

The polysaccharides, or complex carbohydrates, consist of starches and indigestible polysaccharides, such as cellulose. The indigestible carbohydrates are more commonly thought of as "fiber," a foodstuff which essentially only provides bulk.

It is important to realize that a single food or food product might contain many of these forms of carbohydrates. An apple, for example, contains fructose, starch and cellulose. A piece of apple pie might contain fructose, starch, cellulose, maltose, sucrose and lactose. This does not mean, of course, that these foods are composed of radically different forms of carbohydrates—they merely contain several variations of monosaccharides, all built into different structures. In the digestive process, all of these saccharides will be reduced to their "starting point"—monosaccharides—on their way to the cells through the bloodstream.

Besides fats, proteins, and carbohydrates, the other significant nutrients used by the body are vitamins and minerals. Vitamins are simply organic compounds that the body requires. If you can remain healthy without one of these substances, then it is not a vitamin. Because of this definition, there is sometimes controversy over whether or not a particular substance is really a vitamin.

All nutritionists agree that there are now at least 15 compounds that qualify as vitamins. These compounds fulfill a variety of necessary functions; vitamin K, for example, is essential for blood clotting, while vitamin C is needed to help produce the material that connects cells. Most of the vitamins help the function of the body's enzymes, which are needed for many processes, such as digestion.

Certain minerals are also needed by the body in order to be healthy. We eat about an ounce of minerals each day, most coming in the form of sodium chloride, or common salt.

Minerals perform many functions. Calcium and phosphorus, for example, are needed for the bones and teeth, and iodine is needed for the thyroid gland. Other minerals are needed in very small quantities; these "trace" minerals include copper, iron, magnesium and chromium. Vitamins often require the presence of minerals in order to exert their functions; vitamin A, for example, requires the presence of zinc.

Ironically, many of us don't often think of our bodies as being dependent upon substances such as chromium, while many of us do often think of ourselves as being dependent upon starch. In reality, of course, the opposite is true. We do need a little chromium—and we don't need starch.

Why We Don't Need Starch

Starch supplies caloric energy, but nothing else. Foods that contain starch also contain many vitamins, minerals and proteins, however, so we should not eliminate these foods from our diets. The ideal situation is to eat high-quality, vitamin-filled starchy foods in moderation—blocking with the starch-blocker the starch calories that are not needed for energy.

Many nutritionists have recently urged the public to reduce their intake of fat and sugar, and to increase their intake of high-quality starchy foods, such as whole grains and fresh fruits and vegetables. This is sensible advice, especially considering the fact that the average person eats almost two-thirds of all of his or her calories as fat and sugar.

Whole grains and vegetables are generally more healthful than fats and sugars. Nonetheless, high-starch foods can also contribute to an unhealthful diet, *if these foods are eaten excessively.* If more starch is eaten than is needed to meet that day's energy requirements, the starch will be stored in the body, either as glycogen *or as fatty tissue.* This storage of excess starch as fat is what you want to avoid. Excess fatty tissue is unhealthful and unattractive. If this fatty tissue is the result of eating too many starchy foods, then these potentially health-giving foods have been abused; they have been made, through over-eating, into health-destroying fat.

Starch could, of course, be totally eliminated from the diet, since starch *per se* provides nothing to the body except energy—which can also be provided by other foodstuffs. But the total elimination of starchy foods from the diet would rob the diet of some of its most interesting, delicious and high-vitamin, high-mineral foods. Starch is not only impossible to separate from some extremely desirable foods—such as vegetables, grains, and fruits—but it also very helpful in creating many of the processed foods and recipes that we all like. Gravies, sauces, and prepared mixes, for example, all contain high amounts of starch.

Starch itself, then, is, as a nutrient, neither good nor bad—it is merely unnecessary. If it is eaten in direct proportion to the body's energy requirements, it could be considered a "good" food. If it is eaten in excess—without being blocked by the starch-blocker—it could be considered a "bad" food.

Use of the starch-blocker should help most people to get the utmost good from starchy foods. It will help them receive the health-supporting vitamins, minerals and proteins from starchy foods, while blocking the often unneeded starch calories found in these foods.

How the Body Digests Starch

The body digests starch in much the same way that it digests other foods—starch is broken down by digestive fluids and enzymes in the digestive tract, transformed into glucose, or blood sugar, and sent to the body's cells.

Starch digestion begins in the mouth, where a starch-digesting enzyme, known as salivary amylase, digests starch molecules as they are chewed. However, food is in the mouth such a short time that only an extremely small amount of digestion can occur there. Also, because of various chemical conditions, only digestion of cooked starch occurs in the mouth.

The starch then passes through the esophagus to the stomach, where the digestive fluid called "hydrochloric acid" further breaks down the polysaccharide starch molecules that have already been acted upon by salivary amylase. This same digestive acid, though, stops the action of the salivary enzymes that were swallowed with the starch. This, of course, slows down the overall starch digestion.

The stomach, after a very short time, empties the starch into the first part of the small intestine, the duodenum. *It is in the duodenum that almost all starch digestion occurs.* It is here where large amounts of the starch-digestive enzyme called alpha amylase mix directly with starch. The pancreas, where the enzyme alpha amylase is produced, is situated very closely to the duodenum.

The most simple sugars, such as fruit sugars, are absorbed very rapidly. The more complex sugars, such as milk sugar and cane sugar, are also quickly absorbed.

Starch digestion, though, is somewhat more difficult. The polysaccharide starch, under the influence of alpha amylase and hydrochloric acid, is first changed into compounds called "dextrins," then into maltose, and finally into glucose. Glucose is the simplest form of sugar, the form that is absorbed into the bloodstream.

It is during the transformation of starch to dextrins that the starch-blocker does its job.

The transformation of starch to dextrins always requires the actions of the enzyme alpha amylase.

The alpha amylase enzyme molecule joins with the starch molecule at a place on the enzyme molecule that is called the "active site." The enzyme "recognizes" starch, and then accepts the starch into its "active site." This "recognition" occurs through biochemical reactions that are similar to those of, for example, a protein-formed "anti-body," which is able to "recognize" a foreign substance, such as a virus.

When the starch joins the enzyme, the starch is broken down into dextrins, which are further broken down into maltose, and then into glucose.

But, when the starch-blocker is present, the whole chain of events is altered. When the enzyme "sees" the protein substance that we call the starch-blocker, it combines with the starch-blocker. When this happens, the enzyme becomes inactive. As a result, the starch is not broken down.

The enzymes that have bonded with the starch-blocker continue their travel through the digestive system, and are excreted normally with the other unused food products. The starch, meanwhile is also excreted through the normal eliminative processes.

People occasionally note a slight change in their bowel movements when they use the starch-blocker. This is because the undigested starch often adds bulk to the stool. For this reason, people who suffer from constipation may have favorable reactions to the starch-blocker, similar to those which they might experience if they add a high-fiber food, such as bran, to their diets.

Sometimes, people voice a concern that if the digestive enzyme alpha amylase joins with the "wrong" substance—if it joins with the starch-blocker rather than with starch—that the body will then over-secrete the enzyme. However, this does not happen. The pancreas, which produces alpha amylase, fails to "realize" that the enzyme has not joined with the "real thing." Because the pancreas fails to take note that the starch in the duodenum is not being broken down, extra enzyme is not secreted. Therefore, the pancreas remains apparently unaffected by the use of the starch-blocker.

Other people express concern about the starch-blocker entering the bloodstream, and then traveling throughout the body, another occurrence which simply does not take place. The starch-blocker remains in the digestive tract, and is removed from that system in a very short time through normal bowel movements.

The function of the starch-blocker, then, is really quite simple and limited.

But the starch-blocker can have extremely positive effects. It can block the absorption of unnecessary, "empty" calories—calories that can add the pounds to your frame that you try so hard to keep off.

PART TWO

Discovery, Development, Testing

CHAPTER THREE

Discovery

In 1971, while working on several projects at the University of Miami, we came across a puzzling article in a Venezuelan scientific journal. The article, published in *Acta Scientifica Venezolane,* created no furor in the professional community of biochemists who read it—in fact, it escaped the attention of all but a few of the world's biochemists. But the article intrigued us very much, and was responsible for the beginning of our work with the starch-blocker.

The article was written by Venezuelan biologists who had experienced a strange occurrence during work they were doing on the nutritional aspects of kidney beans. These biochemists were feeding rats a diet composed only of raw kidney beans, and found, to their amazement, that the rats who were being fed this presumably wholesome, nutritious diet of legumes did not thrive, but began to waste away. These test animals eventually gradually died, showing every sign of having starved to death—even though the beans they were eating should have contained enough nutrients to sustain life! Death by malnutrition in animals that were apparently being well fed did indeed pose a riddle.

The Venezuelan incident stimulated our curiosity enough to prompt us to review all of the existing scientific literature on the nutritive aspects of kidney beans.

We found several reports of kidney beans inhibiting the growth of test animals. From these reports, we theorized that perhaps some sort of "anti-nutrient"—an agent that would interfere with normal metabolism—might exist in kidney beans. This anti-nutrient, we felt, might prove, upon closer examination, to be a substance that was causing harm to humans. It was possible, we believed, that a similar agent might exist in other edible plant products, and might be responsible for some of the diseases or growth malfunctions that people commonly suffer from. We decided to try to unravel the puzzle.

An important clue to the puzzle was the observation by the Venezuelan scientists that the animals who were wasting away on the raw kidney beans were excreting starch in an undigested form as they lost weight. We inferred, because of this, that there might be something in the kidney beans that interfered with the normal digestive processes that break down starch.

The First Batch!

In the laboratories of the University of Miami, we began to grind up raw kidney beans and make them into an "aqueous extract," or water-based solution. We then studied what role the various components in the extract played in the break-down of starch. What we found was that a substance in the extract appeared to interfere with the action of the primary enzyme that breaks down starch—alpha amylase—an enzyme which, as we have said, is produced by the pancreas and is secreted into the digestive tract.

Our experiments with the kidney bean extracts lay dormant during a year of teaching and research at the University of London.

When we returned to America in 1973, however, to begin directing the Department of Biochemical Research at the Howard Hughes Medical Institute in Miami, we began working on the project in earnest. The Howard Hughes Medical Institute agreed to sponsor our efforts on the projects of our choice for one year, and the kidney bean research was the project we chose to concentrate most of our energies upon. We were determined to solve the puzzle of the apparent anti-nutrient properties of kidney beans. We had not yet, by 1973, conceived of the kidney bean as being the foundation of any sort of weight control formulation. We were, rather, more concerned about it as a possible negative factor in human nutrition.

By 1974, though, it was becoming increasingly obvious that some of the various kidney bean extracts we were working with were harmless, except that they caused weight loss, apparently by interfering with the starch-digesting enzyme alpha amylase. We began to think of the kidney bean extracts as having a positive function.

Toward the end of our first year at the Howard

Hughes Medical Institute, many of the elements of the weight-loss puzzle were falling into place, and the Board of Managers of the Medical Institute was becoming extremely excited over the results of our research. Our successes were apparently brought to the attention of Howard Hughes himself, most likely through George Thorn, M.D., who was Director of Medical Research at the Institute and was formerly a personal physician to Howard Hughes. Howard Hughes, at that time in his life, was traveling throughout the world, but still, it seemed, kept himself apprised of the most promising research project being done by his various businesses and scientific concerns. Just before our first year at the Medical Institute ended, word came down that they wished to renew our appointment for three more years, with a rather substantial increase in support for our work.

Soon the work with kidney beans and starch-blocking became the principal project at the Howard Hughes Medical Institute's laboratories of biochemical research. The project that had begun because of just the curiosity of one man had ballooned into the primary preoccupation of a major research foundation. Over the years, approximately 25 people were involved with the project, though not all were working together at the same time.

During the entire developmental phase of the starch-blocker, over half a million dollars was spent on various aspects of research. Not all of this funding came from any single source, however, and throughout the entire development of the starch-blocker, the concepts and procedures remained our own, and were not purchased by any funding agency nor by any other concern.

This project became increasingly more interesting the longer we worked on it, because the positive possibilities of practical application of the kidney bean extract grew ever more apparent. The kidney bean project overshadowed the other medically-oriented endeavors that we were working on at the time, such as attempting to develop a cure for the relatively rare Tay-Sachs disease, because the bean project seemed to promise the most immediate help for the greatest number of people.

Why the Starch-Blocker Is Important

It is estimated that anywhere between 25 percent to 40 percent of the American public is obese. "Obesity" is defined as being 20 percent over one's correct body weight, or, for example, about 30 pounds overweight on a frame that should be carrying only 150 pounds. Even more Americans, of course, are slightly to moderately overweight, and an extremely high number of people in the totol population are in constant battles with their weights even though they may stay within reasonable weight ranges.

The possibility of making available to the average person a truly effective weight loss formulation, then, was extremely exciting. We realized, as we were working on this formulation, that the starch-blocker had the potential of being one of the most beneficial discoveries ever made. This claim, we sincerely believe, is not exaggeration, but a simple statement of fact. The condition of overweight can be seriously damaging to health, and this condition has, until now, been unsuccessfully addressed by nutritional researchers and the medical profession.

Our hopes for the starch-blocker soared during the years between 1976 and 1980, when we conducted the animal experiments with kidney bean extracts. We found, as we've stated, that the starch-blocker was safe and remarkably effective. We found that it was possible, using the starch-blocker, to reduce the weight gain of growing animals, reduce the weight of full-grown animals, and maintain a weight-loss with a relatively high-calorie diet in an animal that had been on a weight loss diet.

By the time we left the Howard Hughes Medical Institute, in order to join the faculty at a large Midwestern university, all of the theoretical research and much of the practical research on the starch-blocker had been completed.

Many important tasks had yet to be accomplished, though. The production methods of the substance had to be improved, so that an extremely pure and active extract could be produced with unvarying regularity. Production also had to be perfected in terms of commercial viability—if the starch-blocker had cost too much to produce, it could never have been made available at a price the average person could afford, and would therefore never have achieved the degree of social benefit that we felt was possible. The starch-blocker also had to be tested in humans, to prove that it was as effective for people as it was for animals. Finally, the starch-blocker had to be presented to the public in a modest, truthful, dignified manner. We had fears of sensationalistic, "yellow journalism" newspapers exploiting this discovery with headlines screaming: "Eat Yourself Sick and Watch the Pounds Melt Away!!" It was, and is, important to us that this substance—which was painstakingly developed according to the strict standards of the scientific community—never become alienated from the community of careful, reasonable researchers and practitioners.

The refining of the production processes was accomplished. We were able to devise production methods that were commercially feasible. These production methods were also sufficiently refined so that a product could be made available at an affordable price.

The history of the starch-blocker, then, has been a fairly long one, marked by careful scientific investigation in the library, laboratory and clinic. The long, careful effort that went into the development of the starch-blocker was certainly worthwhile, since it resulted in a truly valuable nutritional aid for special dietary use.

CHAPTER FOUR

Development of the Starch-Blocker

At one point in our investigation of the starch-blocker, we had given up. In mid-1975, with a sad, sinking feeling of disappointment, we had abandoned the starch-blocker project. After several months of testing the starch-blocker on rats, we had decided that this substance would never be of use to humans—that it was merely a biological curiosity, one of millions of examples of medical minutiae that are intriguing, but of no practical value. Dismantling the project, we had begun to empty row after row of cages, until our large central laboratory at the Howard Hughes Medical Institute was devoid of any signs of this research effort, which had only recently seemed so laden with promise.

Abandonment of the project had been discouraging to a rather large group of us who had become feverishly involved with the endeavor; this group included many student volunteers from the nearby University of Miami and some of the directors of the medical institute. For months, we had been fascinated by the project, sometimes getting so carried away with it that we had worked around the clock. Scientists who feel that they are on the doorsteps of major scientific break-throughs tend to become fixated upon their work, even obsessed with it, so alluring are the lights at the ends of certain tunnels.

We had become enthralled with the possibilities of the starch-blocker because it had proven to work so well when added to starch-digesting enzymes in test tubes. We had been hopeful, even expectant, that the substance would work equally as well in the digestive system of living animals.

But when we had administered it to rats, it had not fulfilled our expectations. We had done a series of several experiments, feeding the starch-blocker to growing rats, and to rats who had been on a weight-loss diet and were again being allowed to eat freely. Some of the rats in these experiments had been fed a diet containing an average amount of starch, and some had been fed relatively high amounts of starch.

As we had expected, the weight of the growing rats on the starch-blocker had been less than that of a control group of rats who had not been fed the starch-blocker; the rats on starch-blocker had gained about 10 percent less weight as they had matured. We also found, unsurprisingly, that rats that had been on a weight loss diet, and were then given starch-blocker and allowed to eat normally, had gained less weight than a control group that had not been fed the starch-blocker. The difference in weight gain in these two groups was about 11 percent. Another expected outcome was that rats on starch-blocker who had been fed a diet high in starch remained the most underweight of all animals tested.

Why, then, if the weight of the rats had been successfully controlled, were we so disappointed? Why had we given up on the project?

We had given up on the starch-blocker project because such *large amounts* of the substance had been needed to attain our results. If equivalent amounts were to be used for humans, allowing for the weight difference between rats and people, then very heavy doses would have been required to help people control their weights. Weight control could have still been achieved, but people would have had to have spend hundreds of dollars per month on the starch-blocker!

This high cost would have severely limited the ability of most people to use the product. Some people could have afforded it, but this relatively small market for the product would not have justified the great expense of developing it.

Therefore, the rats had been taken off the substance, the cages had been used for other experiments, and we had begun to shift our attention to other projects, even though none of them had fired our imagination as much as had the starch-blocker.

How We Developed the Starch-Blocker

When we abandoned the project, we were certain that we had produced as potent a starch-blocker as was possible. It was not for lack of a high-quality product, we knew, that the experiment had failed. If that had been the problem, we would have returned to the test tubes to perfect our product.

We had first begun trying to produce a pure, potent product soon after we had begun working on the starch-blocker project.

As far back as 1971, we suspected that the substance in the kidney beans that blocked starch utilization was reacting with the starch-digesting enzyme alpha amylase. It made sense to assume that the starch-blocker worked by interfering with the common actions of alpha amylase, simply because alpha amylase is by far the most important substance in the body that is used to digest starch. Therefore, we tested hundreds of different substances derived from kidney beans, mixing them with alpha amylase, to see if they would have any effect on this enzyme.

Deriving all of these hundreds of different substances from the kidney beans was laborious work. First, we had to grind up large batches of kidney beans, then add water or another liquid to them. Then we stirred the mixture to help remove the large particles from it. After this, we strained the mixture, or "slurry," through a screen, to remove even smaller solid particles. Next came a series of processes involving "chromatography," which involves separating the liquid slurry into the various combinations of molecules that compose it. This is done by adding chemicals which contain an "affinity," or ability to attract, different molecules. We collected the various molecular components, or "fractions," in test tubes, and dried them into hundreds of different kinds of powder.

These various powders were then added to the starch-digesting enzyme alpha amylase.

We found that only one of the fractions from the kidney beans was responsible for stopping the normal function of alpha amylase. This fraction was a protein, which we named "phaseolamin." We created this name by combining "phaseo vulgaris," which is the Latin botanical name for kidney beans, with "am," an abbreviation for "amylase," and "in," an abbreviation for "inhibitor." This technical name is what the starch-blocker is called in the scientific literature, and this name is how the starch-blocker is officially registered, with "Dr. John Marshall" listed as discoverer of the substance.

We had, therefore, extracted from a complex biological entity—the kidney bean—a very specific component. This search, which had taken over a year, had been like finding a needle in the haystack.

We still had our biggest job ahead of us, however. We had to find out exactly *what* the "needle" from this "haystack" would do. And we had to find out how well we would do it.

Disappointment

We began adding the protein that we had isolated to alpha amylase. We did this in a series of test tube experiments, or, as scientists say, "in vitro." We found that the protein was most active in a "pH of 6," or in an acid-alkaline balance that is very similar to that found in the digestive tract. We also found that it was best able to interfere with the starch-digestion of alpha amylase at a temperature of 98.4° Fahrenheit, which, of course, is extremely close to the normal temperature of the human body.

It was no surprise to us that the starch-blocker protein was most active in conditions similar to those found in the digestive tract. We had presumed all along that this very interesting ability of the kidney bean to inhibit normal digestion was a survival mechanism in the plant, so we did not believe its strong activity in an atmosphere resembling digestion was a mere coincidence. The starch-blocker that was in kidney beans, we felt, was like the thorn that protects a rose, or the shell that protects a nut. It is simply a protective mechanism that happens to be an enzyme. In fact, the starch-blocker is not even the only protective enzyme-inhibitor found in nature. Digestion inhibitors are found in other plants; the soy bean, to name one, contains a protein that inhibits the action of an enzyme called trypsin. Even the human body contains enzyme-inhibitors—the pancreas, for example, which is where most enzymes are made, secretes certain enzyme-inhibitors that keep its enzymes from "digesting" each other—and even the pancreas itself! Protective mechanisms like these are found throughout nature.

We believe that the enzyme-inhibitor in kidney beans is most effective as a protector against insects, rather than as a protector against larger animals. It is quite hard to say, of course, how a bug "knows" not to eat raw kidney beans. We do know, however, that insects have a tendency to avoid substances that are not nourishing to them. We also can presume that insects that do eat kidney beans may not continue to thrive in the vicinity of a field of kidney beans, for lack of adequate nourishment.

We were able to duplicate in test tubes the conditions resembling those of normal digestion quite easily, merely by controlling factors such as the degree of acid/alkaline balance, temperature, presence of other common chemicals, etc. These "*in vitro*" experiments showed us that the protein we had isolated was indeed very capable of attracting alpha amylase, and thereby keeping it from doing its normal job of digesting starch. The test tube experiments led us to expect great success from the starch-blocker when it was applied to rats. We felt that a small amount of it would block most or all of the starch calories that the animals would normally digest. So of course we were quite disappointed when such large quantities of the starch-blocker were needed to accomplish this task.

We thought that because large amounts had been needed for rats, the substance was unlikely to ever become a commercially viable product. It was at this point that we gave up trying to develop the starch-blocker as a product that could be used for mass consumption, and returned to study it on only a small scale, for the sake of pure scientific curiosity.

Ironically, this small-scale study of the product as a mere biological oddity provided us with a great breakthrough—one which put us back on the track of starch-blocker development with more excitement than ever, and one which paved the way to creation of a substance that we are now certain can help many millions of people.

Breakthrough!

Scaled-down experiments were done in which we studied the activity of the starch-blocker when it was mixed in test tubes with enzymes of various animals.

This work went on for many months, with several interesting, if unsensational, facts emerging. During one phase of the experiments, though, we mixed the starch-blocker with enzymes from a rat. Although enzymes from many animals, and also humans, have previously been used in test-tube experiments with the starch-blocker, no enzymes from rats had been used. The only testing with rats had been with live animals, and these tests, of course, had proven so disappointing that we had abandoned our full-scale research.

To our amazement, though, very little happened when a normal amount of the starch-blocker was added to a test tube containing rat enzymes. We tried the experiment several more times, and still very little reaction occurred.

When an equal amount of this exact same starch-blocking material was mixed with enzymes of animals other than rats, however, excellent results were achieved. We mixed it with enzymes from cats, mice, guinea pigs, humans, and several other species, and the product worked very effectively!

We therefore concluded that, for some unexplained reason, the starch-blocker simply is not effective in reasonable quantities on enzymes of rats. Some peculiarity in rat enzymes makes them so resistant to the starch-blocker that large amounts of it are needed to attain results.

We decided, then, that the starch-blocker might never be effective in rats, but that it might still be highly effective in humans!

With a keen sense of expectancy, we returned to the main laboratory and began preparing experiments that would involve not rats, but mice.

The mice experiments were highly successful, and once again we began work on the project with great enthusiasm. After several more years of hard work, we had developed a product that we were certain would be safe and effective in humans.

The laboratory experimentation days of the starch-blocker were over!

CHAPTER FIVE

How We Know the Starch-Blocker Works

The time had come to study the effects of the starch-blocker on humans. We had become certain, through our many animal tests, that the substance was absolutely safe, and we had every reason to believe, based upon what we had seen it do for animals, that it would also be quite effective as a weight-loss aid for people. But we were not absolutely positive it would be effective. In science, one is never certain of the effectiveness of any substance until it has proven itself to work in carefully controlled studies.

Finding the correct situation in which to test the substance was rather difficult. The study would have to be done carefully and systematically. Furthermore, it had to be conducted with a group of people who were willing to adhere to the fairly strict parameters of the study's protocol.

We realized, after some consideration, that the best way to study the effects of the starch-blocker would be to apply it to a group of persons who were already members of a weight-loss clinic. It was important, in order to establish scientific credibility, and in order to be sure the substance was administered properly, that the clinic be directed by a medical doctor. A medical doctor's metabolic expertise and experience with controlled studies would be necessary in order for us to be sure the study was conducted in a meticulously well-organized manner. The study, we realized, would have to be replicable and verifiable in order to demonstrate that the starch-blocker was an effective product.

The weight-loss organization that we finally chose to perform the study was American Weight Clinics, Inc., of Indiana. We decided to conduct the formal study in several central Indiana clinics that were under the direct medical supervision of Dean Elzey, M.D.

By mid-May of 1981, all the details of the study had been worked out, and we were ready to begin.

How the Study Worked

The study, which was conducted throughout the spring of 1981, consisted of comparing the results of a group of clients using the starch-blocker to the results of an essentially identical group who had eaten a similar diet, but had not used the starch-blocker, and had not been able to eat additional starchy foods.

The group using the starch-blocker was selected

from volunteers who were current clients of the clinic. The "control" group of patients, who were on a similar diet, but who didn't use the starch-blocker, was selected from the case history files of the clinic. The members of this control group were selected on the basis of close physical resemblance to the group using the starch-blocker. For example, if a person using the starch-blocker was a 5′5″, 165-pound, 42-year-old female, a person would be selected from the files who was within two years of age, five pounds of weight, two inches of height and of the same sex. The person selected from the files would have eaten a diet almost exactly like that eaten by the user of the starch-blocker, except that this person's diet would have lacked hundreds of calories of starchy foods every day that the use of the starch-blocker was allowed. At the end of the study, the weight loss of both dieters would be compared.

The hypothesis, of course, was that the person eating the extra starch calories, but also taking the starch-blocker, would lose weight equally as well as the person who had not been able to eat any additional starchy foods. We also hoped that the study would prove that the starch-blocker users, who were able to eat many more calories of starchy foods, would be much more happy with their eating regime, and would be better able to stay with the diet.

The Test Group

The group who volunteered to take part in the study was a group of 90 women who weighed between 133 and 249 pounds. Almost all of them had previously tried to lose weight but had been unsuccessful. All of the people in the study were required to have had a recent physical examination, were required to provide a medical history, and had to undergo routine laboratory tests, such as a complete blood count and standard urinalysis. No patients with chronic illnesses, such as diabetes, were allowed to be part of the test.

The patients were, as a rule, quite excited to be part of this study. All of them had heard several lectures on the starch-blocker and were enthusiastic about putting the substance to use in their lives. Many of them were extremely tired of denial-oriented diets, and were very much looking forward to the increased dietary richness and variety that is possible when the starch-blocker is used. All of the clients realized that they would have to stick closely to the requirements of the study in order for it to be statistically meaningful, and were quite willing to do so.

When the study began, on May 26, 1981, the clients were advised to eat a Base Diet of 500 calories per day of non-starchy foods, mostly high-protein foods. In addition to this Base Diet, they were allowed to eat a certain amount of starchy foods, along with their starch-blockers.

The Base Diet was composed of three meals per day, each consisting of a 3½ ounce portion of protein, a ½ cup serving of vegetables, and a small portion of fruit. The protein could consist of meat, milk or eggs, but clients were advised to use low-calorie protein foods, such as chicken or lean meat or skim milk.

The starchy foods that were eaten in addition to this

Base Diet were added gradually over a four week period. The starchy foods were added gradually, so that we could tell if only a certain amount of starch was being blocked by the starch-blocker, rather than all starch. We presumed that all starch that was eaten would be blocked by the starch-blocker, as it had been in the animal studies, but we could not be certain until we had conducted a careful study with humans. During the first week, clients ate only one extra starchy food per day, adding about 120 calories to their daily diet. In the second week, they ate two starchy foods per day, adding 270 calories. In the third week, they ate three additional starchy foods daily, adding 320 more calories to their Base Diet of 500 calories. In the fourth week, they ate four starchy foods every day, adding 470 calories to the Base Diet, for a total of 970 calories per day.

After the formal four-week study was completed, many of the dieters added even more starchy foods, creating a diet of 500 non-starch calories and 700 starch calories, for a total of 1,200 calories.

The starchy foods that they were advised to eat included popcorn, spaghetti, rice, macaroni, bread, oats, mush, grits, corn, peas, potatoes, parsnips, navy beans and lentils. A number of inviting recipes were suggested to the clients, including both starchy recipes and low-calorie, non-starchy recipes.

The patients were advised to take one starch-blocker tablet with each meal, and to break the tablet in half for all small starchy snacks. Very accurate and careful diet diaries were kept by all patients.

There were no significant problems or complications

during the study. A few of the patients dropped out of the study, but that always occurs during testing. Some patients moved out of the area, or were unable to come to the clinic for weighing and physical testing as often as they were required to. Others were simply unwilling to stay with the prescribed diet, because of the lack of motivation to lose weight. Still, there were fewer drop-outs with this program than with other diets offered by the clinic, probably because the diet was easier than other diets.

At the conclusion of the study, approximately two-thirds of the clients were still actively involved. We were able to include 36 clients in the analysis of the formal study; some of the clients who remained active in the study were not considered viable for statistical analysis. One client, for example, lost 18¼ pounds in one week, which put that client beyond the boundary of the acceptable standard deviation from the norm. Other clients reported straying significantly from the recommended diet, which made their weight-loss results meaningless in the analysis of the formal study. By July, the formal study was completed, and the statistics were ready for analysis.

The results were exciting! The starch-blocker had enabled the clients eating almost 1,000 calories per day to lose as much weight as their counterparts on a 500-calorie per day diet. On the average, they had even lost slightly *more* weight than the control group!

The weight losses in many cases were quite dramatic. Of the 36 people analyzed in the 28-day formal study, there were ten cases of weight loss of 15 pounds or more, and 25 cases of weight loss of ten pounds or more. In the control group, which had eaten about half as many calories as the starch-blocker group, there only six cases of weight loss of 15 pounds or more, and only 20 cases of weight loss of ten pounds or more. In the starch-blocker group, there were seven cases of a weight loss of 17 pounds or more, and in the control group, there were only three cases of a weight loss of 17 pounds or more. In the starch-blocker group, there was only one case of a weight loss of five pounds or less, and in the control group, there were three cases of weight losses of five pounds or less.

Clearly, the starch-blocker group, although they ate almost twice as much, were "better losers" than the control group!

But there was a factor that pleased the directors of the study even more than the weight losses of the group taking the starch-blocker, and that was the psychological reaction of the starch-blocker group.

An almost universal response to a strict weight loss diet is one of feeling deprived, empty and sometimes resentful. Once dieters endure these feelings for a few weeks, they're ready to replenish their feelings of emotional well-being with a dozen doughnuts and a quart of chocolate milk. This predictable gastronomic splurge accounts for the "yo-yo effects" in dieters; "fat-thin-fat-thin."

This need for fulfilling denied desires never emerged among the starch-blocking clients, though! The people who used the starch-blocker, and were able to eat a satisfying array of starchy foods without gaining weight, felt as psychologically strong at the end of the diet as they had at the beginning. In fact, many of them experienced more of a feeling of control over their lives than they had for many years, because they felt they had gained a powerful ally in their ongoing war against weight. Many dieters also reported that planning and cooking meals for their families had been made much easier because of their use of the starch-blocker, which allows more dietary variety.

Because of the relative easiness of weight loss experienced with the starch-blocker group, and because no dieters had experienced negative effects, many of the dieters using the starch-blocker chose to continue the weight-loss phase of the program beyond the four weeks of the study. As a group, they increased their intake of starch to 700 calories per day, giving them a total caloric intake of 1,200 calories. As we assumed, this extra addition of calories did not affect the dieters' rates of weight loss. Because most all of the additional starch calories were being blocked, the end result of the extra caloric intake was essentially equal to one of eating no extra calories.

The 1,200 calorie daily diet seemed to be even more psychologically satisfying than the diets composed of fewer calories. The more people were able to eat, it seemed, the more satisfied they felt, even if the calories they had eaten had not been processed.

Dr. Elzey's Reaction

Dr. Elzey, medical director of the study, was very pleased with its results. Prior to the study, he had been hopeful of positive results, but had not abandoned his good scientist's natural skepticism. "I knew it should work," he said recently, "but I didn't know if it *would* work.

"I had been impressed with the concept of the starch-blocker when it was first explained to me," said Dr. Elzey, "because the scientific reasoning behind it seemed very sound, and the animal experiments appeared to have been carefully done. But I still had no proof that the substance would be effective on humans.

"I first realized it was working, though, when we did clinical tests on the patients who were using it. When these patients ate additional starch calories, we saw *no fewer ketones*, the by-products of body-fat burning, in their urine. If starch calories had been undergoing transformation into energy, there would have been less burning of body fat, and therefore fewer signs of burned fat present in the urine. Because urinalyses of these patients showed no change in ketone levels, regardless of how many extra starch calories were eaten in the study, we knew the starch-blocker was indeed blocking starch calories. Even a slight uptake of these starch calories would have lowered ketone levels. This lack of ketone reduction, I realized, was demonstrable proof of what the weight loss statistics also were indicating—that the starch-blocker was keeping food that was eaten from becoming energy and fat."

Dr. Elzey said that he wasn't surprised that no negative effects were noted by clients during the study. "No one expected to see any negative effects, because of the organic nature of the substance, and because of the extensive preliminary animal experimentation that had been done," he said. "I believe the starch-blocker is one of the safest substances a person could possibly take, because it is an organic product with no systemic effects. Its action is to bind with the enzyme amylase in the duodenum, an action that would not be expected to have any negative effects."

What most impressed Dr. Elzey, though, was the emotional reaction of his clients to the starch-blocker program. "All in all, they were a very easy group to work with, because they were largely content with what they were eating. Most of these people had been on restrictive, low-calorie diets before, and they were amazed that they could eat a relatively normal diet and still lose weight. It pleased them very much, and it pleased me, too."

Dr. Elzey was also very gratified by the response of patients using the starch-blocker as part of a maintenance regime. "The people who were the most happy with the starch-blocker were those who reached their goal weights during the study and then began to use the product as part of their maintenance diets. Many people can stand to restrict their diets during a relatively short weight loss phase, but once they reach their goal weights, they want more generous, varied diets. In the past, these more varied diets tended to cause the regaining of all the weight that had been lost. This occurred much less often, though, with the patients using the starch-blocker. They had a significantly greater ability to retain their weight loss.

"The starch-blocker is really at its best in helping people retain their desired weight, or to shave off an extra pound or two," said Dr. Elzey. "Because of this, I feel that there may be a time when the starch-blocker is in every home, serving as an occasional aid to the average, normal-weight person. This may sound far-fetched right now, but in a few years, I think the idea of almost everyone using a little starch-blocker every so often will seem quite reasonable."

The starch-blocker, then, has been proven to work well, and to work safely. It has proven its ability to make weight control inordinately easier.

Results of Starch-Blocker Clinical Trial

Experimental Group (used starch-blocker)							Control Group (similar patient who did not use starch-blocker)						
Patient	Age	Sex	Height	Weight	Loss Week 1	Week 2-4	Patient	Age	Sex	Height	Weight	Loss Week 1	Week 2-4
19.	37	F	62"	180½	20¼	(8, 12¼)	19.	35	F	64"	174	8	(2½, 5½)
20.	55	F	63"	187½	6½	(3¾, 2¾)	20.	54	F	62"	186¼	10¾	(6¼, 4½)
21.	42	F	66"	230	10	(5,5)	21.	42	F	65½"	230	18	(3¾, 14¼)
22.	20	F	69"	249	13¾	(8¼, 5½)	22.	22	F	67"	249	17½	(N.A.)
23.	44	F	62½"	176¾	14¾	(8, 6¾)	23.	No Match					
24.	52	F	71"	208½	18	(11,7)	24.	51	F	68"	198¼	14½	(5¾, 8¾)
25.	25	F	60"	217¾	18¾	(8½, 10¼)	25	26	F	60"	210	15½	(7¾, 7¾)
26.	39	F	65"	244½	18½	(8½, 10)	26.	35	F	66"	237	9¾	(3½, 6¼)
27.	41	F	62"	182¼	9½	(4, 5½)	27.	42	F	62¾"	186½	8	(3¼, 5¼)
28.	26	F	65"	198½	15	(4¼, 10¾)	28.	24	F	64"	201	13¼	(6½, 6¾)
29.	33	F	68"	205½	20½	(11, 9½)	29.	34	F	66"	197	17	(6¼, 10¾)
30.	32	F	62"	199	15	(5¼, 9¾)	30.	33	F	61"	198	6½	(N.A.)
31.	42	F	65½"	217	9½	(¾, 8¾)	31.	39	F	67"	215	11¾	(6¾, 5)
32.	32	F	66½"	184¾	7¼	(3¾, 3½)	32.	No Match					
33.	25	F	63"	179½	12¼	(¾, 11½)	33.	28	F	62"	187¼	14½	(7¾, 6¾)
34.	44	F	70"	236¾	13½	(1¼, 12¼)	34.	45	F	69"	234½	3	(-¼, 3¼)
35.	50	F	62"	180½	6¾	(4, 2¾)	35.	51	F	64"	181¼	13	(8, 5)
36.	36	F	64"	221	6	(1¼, 4¾)	36.	22	F	65"	221	12½	(3, 9½)

Results of Starch-Blocker Clinical Trial

Experimental Group (used starch-blocker)							Control Group (similar patient who did not use starch-blocker)						
Patient	Age	Sex	Height	Weight	Loss Week 1	Week 2-4	Patient	Age	Sex	Height	Weight	Loss Week 1	Week 2-4
1.	39	F	63½"	175	7½	(5¾, 1½)	1.	44	F	63"	178½	2¾	(-1¾, 4)
1.	39	F	63½"	175	7½	(5¾, 1½)	1.	44	F	63"	178½	2¾	(-1¾, 4)
2.	44	F	67"	186½	17½	(7½, 10)	2.	48	F	66"	196½	16¾	(6, 10¾)
3.	34	F	66"	178½	12½	(5½, 7)	3.	35	F	65"	188	10¼	(2¼, 8)
4.	53	F	62"	147¼	10¾	(5¼, 5½)	4.	53	F	62"	147¼	10	(N.A.)
5.	35	F	65"	141	9½	(2¾, 6¾)	5.	32	F	65"	151	11	(5¼, 5¾)
6.	51	F	65"	142½	10¾	(7, 3¾)	6.	50	F	66"	152	7¾	(2, 5¾)
7.	44	F	62"	164½	8	(-¼, 8¼)	7.	No Match					
8.	55	F	64"	162	12½	(5½, 7)	8.	50	F	62"	160	10¼	(5, 5¼)
9.	56	F	61½"	136½	12	(5¾, 6¼)	9.	57	F	61½"	135½	14	(N.A.)
10.	43	F	61½"	161½	7	(4, 4)	10.	46	F	61"	164	11¾	(3, 8¾)
11.	55	F	64"	146	4¾	(2¾, 2)	11.	55	F	65"	146½	8¾	(2½, 6¼)
12.	67	F	63"	170	12¾	(4¾, 8)	12.	65	F	65"	173¼	6¼	(¾, 5½)
13.	43	F	63½"	156½	9½	(5¼, 4¼)	13.	40	F	62"	160½	4¾	(N.A.)
14.	59	F	65"	181½	12½	(7¾, 4¾)	14.	59	F	64"	180	18¼	(8, 10¼)
15.	50	F	67"	148½	15½	(5¼, 10¼)	15.	48	F	67½"	145¾	13½	(7¼, 6¼)
16.	42	F	66"	155	11½	(9¾, 1¾)	16.	47	F	67"	166½	12½	(4¾, 7¾)
17.	35	F	66"	207½	12¼	(5¾, 6½)	17.	33	F	64"	211¾	6	(3¼, 3)
18.	21	F	62¾	232¼	17½	(N.A.)	18.	No Match					

PART THREE

How the Starch-Blocker Can Help You

CHAPTER SIX

How to Use the Starch-Blocker

Virtually all diet books, sadly, are the same. They're all crammed with the same lame promises, the same gimmicks and the same flimsy word-games. Virtually all of them, in our opinion, are thinly disguised descriptions of fad diets that take advantage of the desperation of overweight people. Almost every diet book ever printed claims the diet that is being promoted causes weight loss: (1) quickly, (2) without hunger, (3) permanently, and (4) while letting you eat heavily.

Although the starch-blocker weight loss program will probably come closer to fulfilling these four promises than any other weight-control program that has thus far been offered, you will find no such bold, bald claims of instant, easy success in this book. In fact, we believe it would be an insult to your intelligence to tell you that getting your weight exactly where you want it, and keeping it there forever, can be done with absolutely no difficulty.

We believe that self-styled diet gurus, like other "carnival barkers of the medical midway," generally adhere to a fundamental law of salesmanship: the weaker the product, the wilder the claims. The fatal flaws of the denial-oriented diets, therefore, have caused a multitude of diet promoters to promise easy achievement of a pie-in-the-sky impossible dream.

Our weight control program, howevers, offers actual fulfillment of realistic wishes to people who are willing to work for their goals.

If you try our program, we will promise you nothing more, and nothing less, than the best chance you have had yet, if you are careful and diligent, to take charge of your body's fat-storage.

The starch-blocker weight control program is not terribly hard to follow, and can be quite successful. Because it employs the most significant breakthrough ever made in the field of weight-loss dieting—use of the starch-blocker—it is actually much simpler to follow than the denial-oriented diets that make such grand claims about their easiness. And it certainly appears to be more effective than these diets. Nonetheless, if the starch-blocker weight control program is not approached with reasonableness and restraint, our program may be of only limited help to the dieter.

The major advantage of our program—use of a substance that blocks starch calories—can be made into the major pitfall, *if the dieter is indulgent and uninformed.* If the dieter falsely assumes that the starch-blocker is a "magic potion," a pill-shaped panacea that will do all the work, then the dieter is asking for trouble. The starch-blocker *must* be used as part of an overall health-building regime. We refer to this regime as the "starch-blocker weight control program." This weight control program includes taking the starch-blocker exactly as recommended, engaging in a regular agenda of exercise, carefully regulating the food that is eaten, and working on the emotional aspects of compulsive eating.

This, obviously, is not a get-thin-quick through-gluttony regime. The starch-blocker weight control program will work amazingly well for those who employ it properly. But it will work only moderately well for those who wish to dedicate their lives to decadence and indulgence.

The starch-blocker weight control program consists of two phases: the weight-loss phase, and the weight-maintenance phase. These two phases, when properly carried out, can end your weight problem forever.

How To Take the Starch-Blocker

People are accustomed to being able to use various pharmaceutical and over-the-counter products in an essentially careless manner—many of us simply do not follow the directions printed on the label of the bottle. Often, this casual attitude toward use-procedures does little to impair the power of the product. It is, for example, hard to misuse an aspirin. *If dieters are careless about how they use their starch-blocker tablets, however, the tablets will not work.* If the starch-blocker tablets are not taken in the recommended manner, there is no point in taking them.

Fortunately, the "recommended manner" is extremely simple—it consists of nothing more than taking the starch-blocker at the same time starchy foods are eaten. As we stated before, the starch-blocker will be active in the digestive tract for only a short time, which we estimate to be about 90 minutes. Ninety minutes is the approximate length of time that it takes most foods to travel from the mouth through the small intestine. The starch-blocker, then, can be expected to move through the digestive tract with the foods it is taken with. Therefore, the starch-blocker must be taken with any foods that one hopes to block the starch calories of. If it is taken one hour—or even 30 minutes—prior to the eating of starchy foods, it can be expected to, for the most part, *precede* these starchy foods in their transit through the digestive tract and therefore have little or no effect upon them. If it is taken 30 minutes to an hour after starchy foods are eaten, it can be expected to *follow* the starchy food through the digestive system, and exert little or no effect upon the conversion of these starchy foods to calories, and then to fat. The starch-blocker tablet, even when it is totally dissolved, occupies only a relatively few inches of cubic space in the digestive system at any one time; particles of it do not become simultaneously widely dispersed throughout the entire digestive tract.

Because the starch-blocker will travel through the digestive system as quicly as any other food, and then be gone, it does no good to take, for example, two or three tablets in the morning, with the expectation that their effects will last all day.

We can not overemphasize this very simple rule: *take your starch-blocker with your starchy foods.*

The best time to take the starch-blocker is from 5 minutes to immediately before a meal.

The tablet should not be chewed, because it may be slightly deactivated if it is excessively exposed to the acid found in the stomach. The tablet should be swallowed with water or any other liquid.

We have no reason to believe that any food, drug or beverage will deactivate the starch-blocker, so there is no need to worry about the neutralizing effects of any food, beverage or medication that is taken with the tablet. The starch-blocker does not have to be taken on an empty stomach, and it does not have to be taken at any special time of day—any time that starchy foods are eaten is the appropriate time to take the starch-blocker.

The starch-blocker can, of course, be taken with starchy snacks. If a snack contains only 50 grams of starch, a starch-blocker tablet can be broken in half, since each tablet eliminates the calories from 100 grams of starch. However, a very starchy meal, containing more than 100 grams of starch, would require more than one tablet to block most all of the starch calories.

Other than knowing that the starch-blocker must be eaten at almost exactly the same time as starch is eaten, the dieter must be absolutely aware of another very important fact. This fact is: *the starch-blocker will affect no foods other than starch.* If the dieter embraces the fallacy that the starch-blocker is an enchanted wonder-pill that will eliminate all calories from all foods, the dieter's waistline may soon balloon.

The starch-blocker, as we have said, blocks starch calories and nothing else!

Dieters must realize that many starchy foods also contain calories from fat and sugar and protein, which the starch-blocker will not affect. A big, doughy cinnamon roll, for example, may have about 100 starch calories in it, but it will probably also have an additional 150 calories of sugar, perhaps another 50 calories of fat, and even some protein calories. Dieters gorging on cinnamon rolls while mitigating their guilt by taking starch-blocker tablets are just kidding themselves. Even if you have blocked all the starch calories from a cinnamon roll, it is still a fattening food.

Other starchy foods may not contain such heavy amounts of non-starch calories, but may still have dozens of extra fat and sugar calories. Many breads, for example, contain some calories from sugar and protein, and any bread with butter on it will contain fat calories. Corn flakes, for another example, may be almost all starch, but the sugar, milk and fruit that may be served with them will contain many non-starch calories. No food is 100 percent starch. Even most foods that are commonly thought of as starchy foods actually derive some of their calories from non-starch components.

Dieters should also be aware that many foods we do not think of as being particularly starchy, such as, for example, beets, actually contain significant amounts of starch. All foods that come from the plant kingdom contain some amount of starch, even though this starch may be "hidden." Therefore, dieters may choose to use the starch-blocker during meals that seem to be "non-starchy."

A list of starchy foods is included in the chapter entitled "The Starch Blocker Diet."

All dieters, if they wish to use this program successfully, must keep in mind the two simple rules we have just stated: (1) *Take the starch-blocker at the same time starch is eaten,* and (2) *Do not expect the starch-blocker to block calories from any food component other than starch.* If these rules are followed, each dieter should be very happy with this powerful new weapon in the "war on weight."

Taking It Off: The Weight-Loss Phase

Dieters all seem to lose weight *fast*—not tomorrow, not even today, but yesterday! The primary reason for this, we believe, is because, until now, all diets have been painful experiences which people have wanted to conclude as quickly as possible. The secondary reason, we feel, is simply that no one wants to be overweight a day longer than necessary. Unfortunately, most fast weight loss diets, known as "crash" diets, create in dieters an emotional, and often physical, need to overeat once the diet ends. This accounts for the "yo-yo effect" that is so common in dieting—five pounds lost are replaced by ten pounds gained.

The starch-blocker weight control program, we believe, will enable this yo-yo effect to be banished forever from the lives of dieters. This will happen with the starch-blocker weight control program because *even during the fast weight loss phase, there will be little sense of deprivation.*

This assertion of little deprivation is an all too common claim. You have no doubt heard it before. All of the promoters of denial-oriented diets maintain that their diets avoid feelings of deprivation, generally because of the use of some little gimmick that they have created. The gimmick may be something as simple as eating slowly, spreading one's food all over the plate, eating from small dishes, or eating lots of low calorie foods, such as celery or diet soda. Sometimes the presumed lack of deprivation is claimed to stem from a more harmful type of gimmick, such as use of pharmaceutical stimulants or caffeine. Promotors of "fasting" weight loss programs claim that total fasts do not cause hunger. Still other diet gurus claim that "metabolism-fooling" techniques, such as eating only meat—or eating foods in certain combinations—overcome hunger and a sense of deprivation.

None of these techniques, in our opinion, truly help dieters to avoid that gnawing sense of deprivation.

None of these mind-tricking and body-fooling schemes seem to really fool most dieters. People don't need master's degrees in nutrition to know when their stomachs are empty.

The starch-blocker substance is the first dietary innovation ever developed that offers dieters a safe, dependable method for eating a satisfying diet and still losing weight. The starch-blocker is the first fast weight control substance that can be used as part of a weight loss program *which will not end in a binge of overeating*. It is the first weight control substance that can make a fast weight loss diet relatively easy, interesting and satisfying, and therefore a diet that a person can remain on for an extended length of time.

It is our fondest desire that dieters will take full advantage of the basic easiness of the starch-blocker weight control program by losing weight at a moderate rate. Weight can, of course, be lost very quickly with the starch-blocker. The tablet can be used, as we've said, to create an artificial "fast," if the starch-blocker is taken with foods that are almost 100 percent starch. *We do not recommend this.* Going on this type of "crash" diet makes as much sense as living on no-calorie diet soda—it is nutritionally dangerous, an actual physical threat to one's system. A diet of this nature would provide very little protein, and it is possible that muscle tissue could be harmed or that mineral imbalances could occur which might impair the function of the heart. No-protein, prolonged fasts have in recent years been strongly criticized by many nutritionists as being a threat to health.

Another disturbing aspect of using the starch-blocker to create an artificial "fast" is that this kind of dieting is a reflection of compulsiveness. In a very real sense, eating absolutely nothing is just a mirror-image reflection of eating everything in sight—both actions are examples of the same compulsive attitude about food. Both actions are divorced from the normal, daily exercise of one's will and common sense. People who are unable to learn moderation, to let go of the all-or-nothing, feast-or-famine mentality, will have a very difficult time ever conquering their weight problems. They may glean a certain glory from the little weight-oriented melodramas that they produce, direct, and star in, but they will probably never be thin people.

Therefore, we sincerely hope that dieters will use the starch-blocker with a moderate, balanced diet, even during the phase in which they are trying hardest to take off the most pounds. The weight will come off slightly more slowly during a moderate diet than during a "crash" diet, but this weight will be much more likely to *stay* off. A dieter on a moderate weight-loss diet will be learning to be un-compulsive, will be learning how to exercise will power on a daily basis, will be learning eating, shopping and cooking habits that can be carried over to the maintenance phase of the weight control program, and will be learning about the various caloric and starch values of foods. If dieters master all of these skills, they should have no trouble maintaining a desired weight for the rest of their lives, with only occasional use of the starch-blocker!

The moderate diet that composes the weight loss phase of the starch-blocker weight control program will last a different length of time for each dieter. It will last last until the dieter reaches his or her goal weight. At that point, the dieter will shift to the second phase of the weight-control program, the maintenance phase.

If the dieter fails to adhere to the maintenance phase of the program and gains extra pounds, the weight loss phase can again be employed. Otherwise, the maintenance phase can be continued indefinitely. The maintenance phase should be easy for dieters to stick to because of the use of the starch-blocker, which allows relatively heavy eating of starchy foods. Consumption of these starchy foods will make the maintenance phase extremely interesting and taste-satisfying.

The average deprivation-oriented diet, in contrast, usually offers a weight-maintenance phase that is about as interesting as a piece of unbuttered melba toast. Dieters on deprivation-oriented maintenance plans usually fail to stay with their weight-stabilizing regime. The starch-blocker, though, will allow the addition of a rich and wide assortment of starchy foods, thus making lifelong slimness attainable for most dieters.

Foods for Weight Loss

During the studies of the starch-blocker on people who were successfully losing weight, it was found that a great many dieters were able to eat as many as 1,200 calories per day and still lose weight at a rate of between one-half to three-quarters of one pound per day. Almost all were able to lose at least one-third of a pound per day. Of these 1,200 calories, approximately 700 came from starch.

The directors of the clinic that supervised the dieters recommended that the dieters begin their weight control program by eating fewer than 1,200 calories per day, then adding more starchy foods each week.

The starch-blocker weight control program certainly should work, of course, if the dieter begins by eating the full 1,200 calories per day, and does not gradually add starchy meals. Some people may prefer to do this, and we will not discourage them from doing so.

From a strictly scientific standpoint, though, we can not claim that this method—of starting with the full 1,200 calories—has been proven to work, since it has not been tested in large, controlled studies. We have observed this method working in individual cases, but in the world of science, observation of individual cases does not constitute proof.

Whether a dieter starts at the 1,200 calorie per day level, or climbs to that level during a one-month period, results should be approximately the same.

Results should be quite similar through either approach because only the 500 non-starch calories will enter the system. Whether a person blocks seven starch calories per day, or 70 per day, or 700 per day, the result is still that most *all* starch calories for that day have been blocked.

Because eating foods containing about 700 calories per day will probably be more enjoyable than eating, for example, foods containing only seven starch calories per day, many dieters will probably prefer to eat more starch calories, and block them with the starch-blocker.

As we have said, a dieter could eat far more starch calories per day than 700, and still block all of these starch calories, if enough of the starch-blocker were taken. But we don't recommend this. We do not want this remarkable dietary innovation to become a crutch for people who wish to be overly indulgent and weak-willed. We wish it to be a tool for people who want to take control of their eating habits, and to learn moderation.

The Base Diet of 500 calories should come primarily from protein, with very moderate eating of fatty foods. Protein, a combination of amino acids that the body uses as "building blocks" for tissue formation, is essential to health. Fats are also essential, but are very high-caloric foods and should be strictly limited. A diet devoid of proteins and fats cannot be considered a healthy diet.

As long as a dieter's body is burning body-fat during weight loss, the dieter will receive the caloric energy stored in that fat. It is not prudent, however, to rely solely upon energy that comes from burned fat. In addition to this fat-derived energy, your body requires essential nutrients, such as vitamins and minerals, that are supplied by food.

The Base Diet of 500 calories that we recommend will supply sufficient nutrients, especially if it is supplemented by all of the vitamins, minerals, fats and proteins that will still be digested from starchy foods. We recommend, though, that the dieter also include vitamin and mineral supplementation as part of the Base Diet. This supplementation may not necessarily be essential, but it certainly makes good sense. Vitamins and minerals contain virtually no calories, and they may immeasurably improve how one feels.

The amounts of vitamins and minerals that people require is a highly controversial subject, with some nutritionists claiming that the average person's diet supplies enough nutrients, and other nutritionists stating that most people live their entire lives with less energy and health than they would have if their diets were supplemented. It is our considered opinion, after much research, that the latter group of researchers is correct—most people, we feel, do not receive enough vitamins and minerals, which are the keys to all of the body's biochemical reactions. Because of these nutrient deficiencies, we believe that our society, as a whole, is less healthy than it would be if all people supplemented their diets prudently. We therefore recommend that people on the starch-blocker weight control program supplement their diets with reasonable amounts of vitamins and minerals.

The Base Diet should also include sufficient liquids. Some dieters become overly concerned about water-weight, even though excess water-weight is really not a common problem at all, compared to weight from stored fat. If there is excessive fluid in the system, it is likely to be there as a result of heavy salt intake, since salt holds water in the body. Salt, therefore, should be reduced, rather than liquid intake. Fluids can be especially helpful during dieting, because elimination of them helps remove the by-products of the burning of body-fat, "ketones."

The 500-calorie per day Base Diet, of course, allows for only a moderate amount of red meat, fish, fowl, butter, oil, milk, cheese, salad dressing, and other foods high in protein, and especially fat. A three-ounce broiled t-bone steak, for example, contains about 190 calories. Three ounces of broiled ground beef contains about 270 calories. One ounce of Swiss cheese contains about 100 calories, a cup of low-fat milk contains about 150 calories. A tablespoon of butter has about 100 calories in it. Three ounces of broiled chicken contains about 120 calories, and three ounces of broiled halibut contains about 150 calories. So, as you can see, the 500-calorie Base Diet is hardly a gourmand's dream!

On the other hand, the Base Diet, when combined with approximately 700 starch calories, can comprise an *interesting, satisfying* daily fare. And remember—this food makes up the weight-loss phase of the diet; the weight maintenance phase is even more rich and pleasing.

We recommend that dieters plan their own Base Diet, using their favorite foods. We have only one strong recommendation for dieters planning their Base Diet, and that is merely to apply common sense in planning. For example, a 500 calorie Base Diet might consist of one piece of pecan pie with ice cream. This would be nutritionally ridiculous, though. A much better Base Diet would consist of an egg for breakfast, a roast beef sandwich and mushroom soup for lunch, fish, green beans and a spinach salad with dressing for dinner, and perhaps some fresh vegetables for snacks. A Base Diet consisting of these foods would supply the following calories: 80 calories from the egg, 120 calories from the roast beef and condiments for the sandwich, 100 calories from the mushroom soup, 100 calories from the fish, 40 calories from the green beans, 40 calories from the spinach salad with a low-calorie dressing, and 20 calories from the vegetables eaten as snacks.

The Base Diet is, of course, a fairly spartan, no-nonsense eating plan. But when use of the starch-blocker is added, a host of interesting, satisfying starchy foods will greatly enliven the Base Diet.

The 700 starch calories that are added to the Base Diet are the equivalent of 175 grams of starch, since four calories are found in every gram of starch. These 700 grams of starch can be added evenly to the three main meals of the day, or used as snacks. Of course, the starch-blocker *must* be taken any time that starch is eaten, or the starch calories will not be blocked.

No meal should contain more than 100 grams, or 400 calories of starch, unless more than one starch-blocker tablet is taken, since one tablet can only block 100 grams (400 calories) of starch.

The dieter should strive, in the selection of the starchy foods that are added to the Base Diet, to choose foods that are as close to 100 percent starch as is possible. This can be done by consulting the "Starch

Content of Foods" chart in the chapter entitled "The Starch-Blocker Diet." A bowl of hot barley cereal, for example, will be about 80 percent starch, while some fruits will be relatively low in starch, compared to their sugar content. Even starchy foods, as we've said, contain calories from non-starch elements, so the dieter should try to eat the starchy foods that have the highest percentage of starch.

Because these extra protein, fat and sugar calories, which are part of starchy foods, will be processed by the body in spite of the use of the starch-blocker, it is difficult to always know exactly how many total calories will be consumed each day by the dieter. The total amount will consist of the 500 calories from the Base Diet, plus however many non-starch calories come from the starchy foods. It is up to the dieter to try to keep the non-starch calories from the starchy foods as low as possible.

Dieters using the starch-blocker who tell themselves that there is no difference between eating a starchy pear and eating a starchy bowl of barley are deceiving themselves. The pear has many sugar calories that the starch-blocker won't affect at all, while the barley has very few.

Dieters should use the "Starch Content of Foods" chart every day. This unique chart is based on data compiled from research.

Dieters on the starch-blocker weight control program will need more than the common charts found in many other books that list only carbohydrate content of foods. These carbohydrate-content charts, which don't define how much of the carbohydrate content comes from starch and how much comes from sugar, are of little value to the starch-blocker diet. A brownie, for example, might contain 150 to 200 calories of carbohydrates, but only about 25 to 40 of these calories will be starch calories. The rest will be sugar calories which the starch-blocker will have no effect upon.

The dieter should strive not only to choose starchy foods that contain few calories from fats, sugars and protein, but should also try to choose foods that are nourishing, interesting and diverse. An exciting assortment of breads, potato dishes, pasta, grains and vegetables can be mixed in a creative, appetizing way, forever ending the boredom and lack of fulfillment that is associated with virtually all of the denial-oriented diets.

The sample Base Diet we mentioned can be greatly enlivened. This Base Diet, you will remember, consisted of—breakfast: one egg; lunch; roast beef sandwich and mushroom soup; dinner: fish, green beans, spinach salad; snack: fresh vegetables. This fairly strict diet can become, with the use of the starch-blocker: breakfast: one egg, toast, hash browns, and a starch-blocker. Lunch: a roast beef sandwich, mushroom soup, curried rice, tapioca pudding and a starch-blocker. Dinner: baked cod, green beans, spinach salad, a dinner roll, noodles, a baked potato, and a starch-blocker. Snacks: vegetables, muffins, and biscuits, each eaten with a half of a starch-blocker tablet.

To a person who has lived for years on denial-oriented diets, this menu probably sounds too good to be true. But this is, of course, quite a realistic approach to weight-loss dieting, one that provides for safer, more permanent weight loss than other approaches previously devised.

And remember: this is still the weight-loss phase of the starch-blocker weight control program. The rich, delicious maintenance phase very closely resembles the average, or even above-average, calorie consumption of most Americans.

As we've said, starch normally accounts for about 25 percent of the calories of the average diet, *and these calories can be basically eliminated, if the starch-blocker is used.* If people using the starch-blocker consciously shift to a higher-starch diet while taking the starch-blocker, the percentage of their diet that never becomes calories can be *even higher!*

Other foods that could be added to the Base Diet of the weight loss phase of the program include a diverse sampling of your favorite foods. Breakfast might include, as part of the Base Diet, fruits, fruit juice, yogurt, nuts, milk, or steak. Breakfast's starchy foods can include hot and cold cereals, certain fruits, all kinds of breads, including toast, rolls and muffins, and various potato dishes. Lunch and dinner starchy foods might include beans, corn, peas, potatoes, yam, barley, biscuits, breads, rolls, macaroni, pizza, noodles, spaghetti, crackers, lentils and certain desserts, such as specially prepared rice and bread puddings, or tapioca.

There are no foods that are "forbidden." "Forbid" is a word one applies to children—it is not a dietary concept we wish to ever hold over the heads of mature, intelligent adults. One must merely use common sense. Why would a person, for example, want to eat one piece of a rich desert, and thereby reach the 500-calorie daily limit for non-starch foods? Any sugary, high-calorie foods that are eaten will have to displace nutritious low-calorie foods, if the weight control program is to work. And if this replacement of nourishing foods with high-sugar or high-fat foods is done regularly, the dieter's energy, mood stability, and possibly even health may suffer.

Alcohol and caffeinated drinks are not restricted from the starch-blocker weight control program, but these drinks must be recognized for what they are. Alcohol is a very high-calorie drink in almost any of its varied forms, and is particularly fattening when used as part of a sugary mixed drink. Even a low-calorie gin-and-tonic contains about 70 calories, and most beers are in the 120-calorie per bottle range. White wine, at 25 calories per ounce, is one of the lower-calorie alcoholic drinks.

Alcohol is also a notorious weakener of will-power and self-control, and could touch off an episode of binge eating. It is also dangerous to the entire system, a destroyer of certain vitamins, and stressful to the liver, kidneys and sometimes the pancreas and stomach. Problems with any of these major organs can create diet-disturbing metabolic imbalances, such as food allergies, indigestion or hypoglycemia.

Caffeine is another substance which can wreak havoc with a diet. Most of the promoters of denial-oriented, calorie-counting diets stress moderate to relatively heavy use of caffeine drinks, such as coffee, tea and caffeinated diet sodas, since these drinks are low-calorie, provide energy, help fill up the stomach, and depress the appetite. What these irresponsible diet-gurus pushing caffeine don't mention, though, is that caffeine elevates the body's energy only temporarily, by stimulating the pancreas, adrenal glands and central nervous system, and then causes a rapid energy plummet when the "high" wears off. This energy drop, of course, can make dieters hungrier and weaker than they had been before their coffee, tea, or diet cola.

Sometimes the energy "crash" from a couple of cups of coffee can be so severe that the dieter feels almost incapable of resisting foods that will bring the energy level back up, and therefore reaches for the foods that most quickly elevate energy levels. These foods are, of course, sugary foods. These sugary foods will cause a similar fast-up, fast-down energy instability, creating a vicious spiral of dependence upon caffeine and sugary foods for rapid energy. This spiral has ruined many diets.

Dieters who manipulate their energy levels with caffeine are playing a dangerous game, one that may well end with an eating binge. The truly serious dieter should try to limit caffeine use to a bare minimum, and will be aware each time that caffeine is used that an energy drop may soon occur. The best way to overcome this energy drop, if it does occur, is to sit down and relax if possible, to eat a high-protein food, and to wait patiently for the energy level to stabilize. Stabilization should occur within 30 to 60 minutes.

Similarly, we do not have any particular admiration for diet sodas—even non-caffeinated ones—or many other artificially-sweetened foods. These highly chemicalized foods may someday be proven dangerous.

When a desire for a sweet food does occur, though, the dieter may be best off by satisfying the urge with a food sweetened by "aspartame," the new sweetener made of natural proteins. This sweetener may well be more conducive to health than highly synthetic sweeteners.

There will, by the way, probably never be a "sugar-blocker," because if sugar were to sit undigested in the gastro-intestinal tract—as starch does when the starch-blocker is used—it would ferment, and cause considerable discomfort.

With the great diversity of starchy foods provided in the weight-loss phase of the starch-blocker weight control program, a dieter should not have a strong need for caffeine or synthetic, no-calorie non-foods. These "make-believe" food products are not needed as crutches with our program. Even during the weight-loss phase, our program provides a satisfying, interesting daily diet.

The Maintenance Phase

Maintenance has always been the disastrous stage of every diet. *Until now!*

The majority of people who have run the gauntlet of weight-loss gimmicks and fad diets have actually succeeded in losing some weight. And they have then succeeded equally as well in *regaining every lost pound.* Often, people gain back more weight than they had initially lost, because of physical and emotional stresses that their diets caused.

Quite clearly, maintaining the weight that was initially lost is the most difficult aspect of dieting. *It is in overcoming this problem that the starch-blocker weight control program is at its best.*

The weight-loss phase of the weight control program, as we have shown, can be quite effective. But it is as a maintainer of desired weight that the starch-blocker is, compared to other diet plans, most effective.

Many other diets can help dieters lose weight as quickly—if not as painlessly—as can the starch-blocker weight loss phase, but no diet we know of can help dieters *maintain* weight losses as well as can the starch-blocker weight maintenance phase. The reason for this, of course, is astoundingly simple: on our weight maintenance plan, *you get to eat more.*

If fact, during the starch-blocker weight-maintenance phase, which goes on indefinitely, you can eat as much as, or even more than, the average person. You can do this because you will be eliminating starch-calories by using the starch-blocker.

As we've shown, most people derive about 25 percent of their calories from starch. If dieters blocked most all of these calories, which can be done with only about three starch-blocker tablets per day, they would, in effect, be living on about 25 percent fewer calories than before. This 25 percent reduction should be sufficient to maintain dieters' desired weights indefinitely, with only reasonable attention paid to calorie counting or food restriction, particularly if people are cautious about the amount of fat they eat.

It is our desire, though, that dieters continue to eat with moderation, prudence and common sense, and gradually *reduce their use of the starch-blocker.* After all, starch calories can also be "blocked" by not eating them in the first place. It is not, of course, unhealthful to continue to use the starch-blocker frequently, but we simply think that people are happiest when they feel the least in need of any particular substance, no matter what it is. People seem to feel most proud of themselves when they accomplish their goals with their own will-power and common sense, rather than with a scientific innovation. Maybe we are just old-fashioned believers in the creed of rugged individualism, but the fact remains that will-power and common sense are needed in every facet of life—they're indispensible!—and if one develops these traits, they can be applied with equal ease to all aspects of living, including one's diet.

We recommend, therefore, that the dieter continue to eat a variation of the high-protein, low-sugar, low-fat Base Diet, along with a variety of interesting, tasty, healthful, starchy foods. During maintenance, more calories can be eaten in both the Base Diet part of the program and in the starchy foods part of the program.

The Base Diet can be expanded to about 1,000 to 1,200 calories per day, or even somewhat more, depending upon one's height, build and degree of physical activity. Another approximately 1,000 to 1,200 daily starch calories can be eaten. This would bring the daily diet's total calories to about 2,000 to 2,400, with about 1,000 to 1,200 of those calories—the starchy ones—being blocked by the starch-blocker. Frequent use of the starch-blocker, therefore, would bring the number of calories processed by the body back down to 1,000 to 1,200.

Most people probably would *not* want to block *all* 1,000 to 1,200 of their starch calories, because the 1,000 to 1,200 calories per day that would be left to live on might not provide enough energy for them, if they are down to their desired weights and are no longer burning stored fat. These people, then, would have to either receive more protein calories from their Base Diet, or take fewer starch-blocker tablets. We recommend that they simply take fewer starch-blocker tablets. As we've said many times, we do not want the starch-blocker to be used to promote overly indulgent eating.

A woman who is average in height and physical activity is generally considered to need about 1,500 to 1,800 calories per day, while a man of average height and physical activity is generally thought to need about 2,000 to 2,400 calories. Of course, there are considerable variances to these "average" needs. We believe that many people, because of metabolic variances, will gain weight even if they eat only the number of calories that weight-charts say they are "supposed" to eat. As a rule, only the individual really knows what his or her caloric needs are, and these needs can vary from season to season and year to year.

There is a simple guide to establishing one's proper caloric intake—if you start to put on extra weight—weight which you can clearly identify as stored fat—then it is time to either reduce your caloric intake, or use the starch-blocker more frequently, or to increase your amount of physical activity. The most sensible thing would be to engage in all three of these strategies.

Some people will need to eat less than the "average" person, because of their metabolic characteristics. About three percent of the general population, and probably about six percent of all seriously overweight people, have clinically diagnosable thyroid problems. Many more people probably have slight thyroid deficiencies, or other glandular imbalances, which require them to eat less food than the average person.

Assuming, though, that the dieter has no substantial metabolic problems, he or she should thrive on the

1,000 to 1,200 calorie Base Diet, eaten with the 1,000 to 1,200 calorie starchy-foods component. This combined Base Diet and starchy-foods component, not all of which, of course, will be processed as calories, should provide a level of food intake that will *satisfy almost anyone.*

For example, this diet might include the following daily foods. Breakfast could consist of two eggs, hash browns, two pieces of toast, a piece of meat, and a glass of orange juice, for a total of about 550 to 600 calories. A morning snack of two pears would add 200 calories. Lunch could be a broiled veal cutlet, broccoli in cheese sauce, tomato juice, and a green salad, for about 450 to 500 calories. An afternoon snack of cream of potato soup would add 140 calories. Dinner would be pan-fried haddock, a baked potato, two dinner rolls with butter, cauliflower in white sauce, a dinner salad with dressing, and tapioca pudding and fruit for dessert, for about 650 calories. An evening snack of a baked apple would add about 100 calories. The total for the day would be about 2,180 calories. If the cauliflower in white sauce, orange juice, cream of potato soup, and piece of meat were eliminated, the caloric intake would fall to about 1,400 to 1,500. If all of the starch calories were blocked, the total caloric intake would drop by about 600 calories, or to about *1,600 calories for the full daily plan and about 900 calories for the reduced plan* (with the cauliflower, orange juice, soup and meat removed).

Once again, this sounds almost *too good to be true.* But it is true. A maintenance diet this rich and diverse is a diet that most people actually *can* maintain! The addition of the starch-blocker, with its calorie-blocking abilities, makes the difference in creating a maintenance plan that can go on, with only a modest effort on the part of the dieter, *indefinitely!*

Dieters using the starch-blocker can, of course, eat foods higher in starch content, and thereby increase the amount they eat without increasing the calories that turn into fat. This probably will not be necessary for most people, though. Even occasional use of the starch-blocker will block enough calories to make the maintenance phase work for most dieters.

If dieters do choose to eat relatively more starchy foods during their maintenance periods, they should try to use balanced, wholesome starchy food products. We recommend that dieters choose their starchy foods from a wide assortment of vegetables and grains. Rather than, for example, eating slice after slice of bread, a dieter should pick his or her starchy foods from an array of potato dishes, rice, cooked grain cereals, cold cereals, lentils and other beans, corn, noodles, pasta, crackers, biscuits, rolls and macaroni. Diversity will keep the diet *interesting,* and will *provide many nutrients.* Dieters should remember that only the starch in starchy foods is blocked—the vitamins, minerals and other nutrients in the starchy foods are digested normally.

We advise dieters to use whole grain products and fresh vegetables, rather than processed grains and vegetables.

Nutritional scientists have proven that whole grain products, such as whole wheat bread or brown rice, are far superior nutritionally to grain products that have been highly processed. Both processed and unprocessed starchy foods respond equally well to the effects of the starch-blocker, but unprocessed foods will provide the body with more of the nutrients it needs, and will provide the fiber that the lower bowel requires for proper function. A dieter has everything to gain and nothing to lose by using whole grains.

Fresh vegetables are preferable to frozen or dried vegetables, and frozen or dried vegetables are preferable to canned vegetables. Fresh vegetables are much more likely to contain all of the food's original nutrients, which can be destroyed during storage. Many canned vegetables contain sugar and salt; sugar is very fattening and salt can cause extra water weight in the body.

Dieters on the maintenance phase of the starch-blocker weight control program should never stop trying to improve their diets.

Learning to eat as healthy a diet as is possible should be a lifelong goal of everyone—not just people with weight problems. It is becoming increasingly clear to health authorities that careless diets, high in sugar, fat, salt and processed foods, are linked to most of our common diseases, including arthritis, heart disease, diabetes and cancer.

Even after dieters conquer their weight problems, they should still try to eat well in order to avoid these tragic degenerative disease conditions, and in order to live life with the energy, joy and stamina that is possible when a careful diet is consumed.

If dieters on the maintenance phase will follow one simple precept—if they will eat to live, rather than live to eat—they will find the maintenance phase easy, and exceptionally rewarding.

Exercise and Weight Control

People gain extra fat by taking in more energy in the form of food than they expend as activity. If people were strenuously active all day long, they could eat virtually anything they wanted. Laborers who work hard all day can easily consume 3,000 to 5,000 calories and not gain weight, because they expend 2,000 to 4,000 calories every day at work. Marathon bicyclists burn up to 10,000 calories per day!

Most people, however, burn far fewer calories through their regular daily activities than do marathon bicyclists. The average office worker probably burns only about 1,000 calories during the day, and even most people who are relative active in their jobs burn off only about 1,500 calories.

It makes good sense for a dieter to try to increase his or her amount of physical activity. If a person goes for a brisk half-hour walk every day, by the end of the week, over 1,000 calories will have been used up, accounting for a weight loss of about one-third of a pound. This caloric use would be approximately equivalent for a dieter to not eating for an entire day. If a person is more active, and exercises energetically for an hour a day, about 3,000 calories will be burned per week, for a weight loss of about a pound. This calorie use would be equal for a dieter to not eating for two or three days! Exercise will not only use up body fat, but will also tone muscles and improve circulation.

We know of no reason why people on the starch-blocker weight control program should not be able to exercise as much as their general physical conditions allow. Anyone who has extra weight to lose will be provided with sufficient energy for exercise through the burning of body fat. No extra fatigue should be noticed, even during the weight-loss phase of the weight control program.

If people reach their goal weights, and then feel exceptionally weak or tired after exercise, it may be an indication that not enough food is being eaten, or that perhaps fewer starch-blocker tablets should be used. If this experience happens only on rare occasions, it probably is not indicative of a shortage of food calories being eaten. If it happens each time one exercises strenuously, though, it probably is an indication that the body needs more food energy than it is receiving. If this is the case, however, there should also be other signs of insufficient caloric intake—most notably, too much loss of weight, causing an appearance of excessive thinness.

Following are a list of activities and the number of calories that each burns up. Our general recommendation to healthy persons is to engage for 30 to 60 minutes every day in an activity that burns up at least 250 calories per hour. People who are elderly, or considerably overweight, or who are in ill health, should consult with their physicians before beginning an exercise program.

Type of Activity	Calories Per Hour Used
SEDENTARY ACTIVITIES, such as: reading, writing, eating, watching television or movies, listening to the radio, sewing, playing cards, typing, miscellaneous office work, and other activities done while sitting that require little or no arm movement.	80 to 100
LIGHT ACTIVITIES, such as: preparing and cooking food, doing dishes, ironing, walking slowly, miscellaneous office work and other activities done while standing that require some arm movement, rapid typing, driving, other activities done while sitting that are more strenuous.	110 to 160
MODERATE ACTIVITIES, such as: making beds, mopping and scrubbing, sweeping, light gardening, carpentry, walking moderately fast, other activities done while standing that require moderate arm movement, and activities done while sitting that require vigorous arm movement.	170 to 240
VIGOROUS ACTIVITIES, such as: heavy housework, bicycling, climbing stairs, dancing, playing baseball, exercising moderately, playing golf, walking fast, bowling, gardening, playing ping-pong.	250 to 350
STRENUOUS ACTIVITIES, such as: swimming, playing tennis, running, bicycling or dancing very energetically, playing football, sawing wood.	350 & more

Exercise can be used as a way to compensate for eating too many calories. A person who eats 250 extra calories at a meal, for example, could take an hour-long walk afterwards to burn up the extra calories.

Exercise should be engaged in during the weight loss phase, and then carried into the maintenance phase of the weight control program. It should become an integral part of everyone's life, just as a prudent diet should. Many people do not have an eating problem so much as they have an exercise problem—they eat with basic moderation but are so inactive that they still gain extra weight. Exercise, which can be made extremely pleasant when one finds the activity with the most appeal, should *always* be considered *an important part* of the starch-blocker program.

The Psychology of Overeating

As important as regular exercise is addressing the emotional makeup of the person who is trying to maintain a desired weight. All too often, emotional problems lie at the root of weight problems.

You will not find in this book a plethora of pithy positive-thinking pep-talks, because we believe that most people whose emotions are causing their overweight conditions need far more than a paragraph of encouragement in order to solve their emotional problems. Many people with strong impulses to overeat need counseling from someone who understands compulsive behavior, and they also need strong support from families and friends. Weight loss clinics are often quite helpful to dieters needing counseling and support. We encourage dieters who are compulsive eaters to either join a reputable weight loss clinic or club, or to seek individual or group counseling. The self-examination occuring during counseling can be an enriching opportunity for growth and exploration, and can, needless to say, solve many more problems than just one's dietary problems.

Our program, though, offers a special psychological benefit all its own. The starch-blocker weight control program can be of *great benefit* to the emotions of the person who has thus far been unable to control his or her eating habits. It is our opinion, after talking to many overweight people, that many compulsive eaters share the trait of feeling essentially *out of control of their lives.* Much of this feeling of lacking control seems to have become centered on their inability to control their weights and eating habits. We believe that the starch-blocker, with its extraordinary ability to give dieters a "helping hand," may help reinvest these people with a sense of control and power. It is our hope that after people learn that they can control their weights, that they will also begin to feel that they can control the other aspects of their lives. These other aspects, such as family or job situations, may have led to their compulsive overeating in the first place.

This regaining of a sense of control may not work for everyone, but it should work for many. Compulsive eaters may find out that they are not nearly as weak as they had thought they were. Many people who feel they can't control their eating habits just need an extra "boost," and *the starch-blocker provides that boost.*

Using the Starch-Blocker

Using the starch-blocker, as we have shown, is not at all difficult. The natural food substance can be used as a nutritional aid in taking off extra pounds, and can be used with relative ease to maintain a proper weight.

Dieters using the starch-blocker need only proper information, a little will-power and perseverance, and the motivation to want to live at a desired weight for the rest of their lives.

CHAPTER SEVEN

How Not To Use the Starch-Blocker

The only way to incorrectly use the starch-blocker is simply to expect too much from the product. If you expect the starch-blocker to block the calories from foods other than starch, or if you expect a tablet taken in the morning to still be active by evening, you will be deceiving yourself about the protection against calories you are receiving.

If, for example, you eat a "starchy" piece of angel food cake with some "starchy" maple-nut ice cream on it, and expect to gain no weight because you are taking the starch-blocker, you are headed for trouble. The cake and ice cream, laden with fat and sugar, will pile the pounds on, despite the fact that the starch calories in these rich foods will be blocked.

Likewise, if you take three starch-blockers in the morning, hoping that the calories from your macaroni and cheese lunch and spaghetti dinner will be blocked, don't be surprised if your bathroom scale has a nasty little surprise for you the next morning! The starch-blocker travels through the digestive tract as quickly as any other food, and will block only the starch calories of the meals it is taken with.

As we showed years ago in laboratory testing, the starch-blocker does not produce short-term or long-term negative effects. It is a totally natural product, one that only aids in nutritionally inhibiting the digestion of starch. As we have shown, the starch-blocker does not even change the enzyme that digests starch—it merely binds with this enzyme. In its purified form, the starch-blocker itself has no effect on organs or tissues, in the body.

However safe the starch-blocker products may be, the fact remains that people can hurt themselves by taking their own "home-made" starch-blocker. This amateur dabbling in a complex production process can have unfortunate results!

On a few occasions during the development of the starch-blocker, in the period before the substance was available to the public, we received telephone calls from people who were sick to their stomachs. These people had heard rumors about raw kidney beans being used in our laboratory to eliminate calories. Some of these people had seen an irresponsible article printed in a sensationalistic newspaper that had made careless and inaccurate references to the work we were doing. These people, for whom a little knowledge had become a dangerous thing, had embarked upon their own efforts to produce a starch-blocker. Most of the people had simply ground up a batch of kidney beans in an electric blender, had mixed the resulting powder with water, had drunk the mixture, and had then hoped for the best! The best did not happen, though—the worst did. Most of the people who had eaten the raw kidney beans immediately began suffering from indigestion, excessive gas in their stomachs, abdominal bloating, diarrhea, and flatulence. They had fallen victim to a factor that nutritional scientists have long been aware of—toxic substances in raw kidney beans.

We had known from the beginning of our research that kidney beans contain certain chemical elements, which are deactivated during cooking, that are toxic to animals and man.

In the production of our starch-blocker, we had learned how to eliminate these toxins from the finished product without reducing the strength of the starch-blocker. Removing these toxins is difficult, and is not a job that can be done in the family kitchen!

We found during our experimentation that small animals could die if they ate a large amount of these toxins, so we were scrupulously careful to remove all traces of them.

Therefore, we offer a strong warning to people *not to grind up and eat raw kidney beans or to use products that have not been prepared according to our techniques*. Anyone who does this is not only risking probable short-term feelings of illness, but may be causing long-term damage to his or her body.

If people try to eat a very small amount of their own ground-up beans or use inferior products in order not to get a heavy dose of toxins, they will find that a small dose of ground-up beans does not contain enough starch-blocker to block very much starch. In order to actually block an appreciable amount of dietery starch, so many raw kidney beans would have to be eaten that the dieter would almost certainly become ill.

So stay away from crude, home-made or improperly made commercial starch-blockers—and stay healthy!

Who Shouldn't Use It

We can not recommend that any person with a special metabolic problem, such as diabetes, use the starch-blocker. We have no specific reason to believe that the substance would have negative effects upon people with such special metabolic problems, but until further research is done, it does not seem prudent that diabetics or people with other similar problems use the starch-blocker without consulting their physicians.

A few people with food allergies may react to beans, and these people should be cautious about using the starch-blocker, since it is derived from kidney beans.

A few people may notice minor bloating, which is sometimes caused by the increased abdominal bulk created by undigested starch passing through the digestive tract. This bloating seems to no longer occur after a few days of using the starch-blocker.

We also recommend that pregnant or lactating women avoid using the starch-blocker. No harmful effects have been observed, and we know of none that might be expected to occur, to either mother or child. Still, this crucial period is a time to err on the side of over-nutrition, if one must err at all. Doctors generally do not recommend that pregnant women, or women who are nursing, undergo a weight-loss during pregnancy—and moderate to regular use of the starch-blocker certainly might cause weight loss. If a pregnant or lactating woman does have a strong desire to take the starch-blocker, we recommend that she consult her physician about it.

Another group that should not use the starch-blocker is composed of people who are already underweight. This group would include people suffering from "anorexia nervosa," the psychological disorder characterized by a condition of extreme underweight and unwillingness to eat. Anorexics, who have a morbid fear of being overweight, and who generally do not perceive themselves as being unattractively and unhealthily thin, may want to use the starch-blocker to further their self-destructive behavior. There is no way to stop them from doing so, just as there is no way to force them to eat. Doctors and family members of anorexics should, however, try to discourage this use. Use of the starch-blocker by people who are moderately underweight should also be discouraged. These people should be encourage to eat, and to not use any products that will aid further loss of weight, whether these products are diet sodas or the starch-blocker.

The world's mass media has made attainment of a reedy, sylph-like figure into, literally, an international fetish. Millions of people, including many with perfectly acceptable weights, yearn to emulate the "starved-look" of fashion models, and will willingly sacrifice their health to achieve this dubious goal. Women, in particular, seem vulnerable to belief in this contrived ideal. Most diet gurus, of course, encourage people not to break away from the concept that thinner-is-better, regardless of the consequences. These gurus' books are crammed with reinforcement of the myth that "as the pounds melt away, all of life's problems will become magically solved."

We would prefer that people learn to accept themselves as they are. The world will be a more reasonable place when people stop measuring their own self-worth by measuring their waistlines. We believe that when and if worship of the Twiggy-look ceases, much of the all-or-nothing obsessiveness about eating will fade away. And when this happens, it would not surprise us at all to see millions of people shed their excess weight and live health-centered, exuberant, *thin* lives.

CHAPTER EIGHT

The Starch-Blocker Diet

The starch-blocker weight control program will probably prove to be the most richly satisfying, exciting diet you have ever been on—because it is not based on denying you the foods you love. Life is simply too short to deny yourself the rewards of dietary pleasure.

The previous diets you may have tried—which were almost certainly based on denial and deprivation—probably failed. They failed because they were too hard to stay on. You will be able to stay on the starch-blocker program, however, because it is a filling, interesting, delicious diet.

Because of the use of starch-blocker tablets, you will *be able to eat more* on this diet than other diets you have tried before. Because the starch-blocker greatly reduces digestion of starch calories, you will be able to eat a wide variety of taste-pleasing starchy foods, but your body will not process, digest and absorb the calories from these foods. You may, therefore, eat reasonable amounts of starchy foods, and create for yourself a daily culinary fare that is as engaging and tasty as it is healthful and low-calorie.

You will still, of course, have to apply common sense and self-control in your eating habits. Because the starch-blocker blocks only starch calories, and not calories that come from fat, sugar and protein, you will have to control your fat, sugar and protein intake. You can not, for example, eat all the chocolate cake and ice cream that your heart desires, because the sugar and fat in these foods will heap pounds of fat onto your body. If you are accustomed to eating high amounts of fat and sugar, as many overweight people are, you will have to change your eating habits to succeed with this program.

Of course, the reduction of starch calories you will derive from the starch-blocker will help you compensate for the overeating of fat and sugar, but this compensation will probably not be sufficient to give you the kind of physique you desire. You can, for example block as many as one thousand starch calories per day, but if you are still eating 2,500 to 3,000 fat and sugar calories each day, you will almost assuredly not lose weight.

If, however, you eat fat and sugar in *strict moderation,* and also use the starch-blocker to block starch calories, *you will almost certainly lose weight.*

Because the starch-blocker eliminates starch calories, you may want to eat a diet that is somewhat higher in starch than the diet you are now eating. You will want to substitute starchy foods for sugary and fatty foods.

If, for example, you like to have a high-fat, high-sugar, deep-fried doughnut for a snack, you may want to substitute for the doughnut a low-fat, low-sugar, high-starch English muffin. An English muffin, lightly buttered with whipped creamery butter and sweetened with apple butter, would be about 225 calories *without* a starch-blocker, containing almost as many calories as a doughnut. But it will only be about *35 calories* if you eat it with half of a starch-blocker tablet! When you compare this 35 calorie snack to a 250-calorie doughnut, you can see how the starch-blocker will help you to lose weight.

It is crucial, though, that you realize the importance of minimizing calories by using techniques such as buttering your food *lightly* with *whipped* butter, and using apple butter instead of sugary jam. If, for example, you ate an English muffin with a starch-blocker tablet, but buttered it heavily with non-whipped butter and coated it with blackberry jam, your 35-calorie snack would become a *320-calorie snack!* You would have added 200 calories of butter (2 tablespoons), and 100 calories of jam (4 teaspoons). If you are careless about sweeteners and condiments, you may as well eat doughnuts.

You must never forget that high-fat foods, such as whole milk, cheese, salad dressings, butter, and many meats, are invulnerable to the effects of the starch-blocker, and so are high-sugar foods, such as desserts, many fruits, and syrups.

If you are to be successful with this great new weight control program, you can not be unaware of the caloric contents of foods, as many people are. We have included in this book lists of the caloric contents of starchy and non-starchy foods, and you should consult this list every day.

Hidden Sugar and Fat

One of the reasons people tend to be unaware of the caloric contents of the foods they eat is because many of the calories in these foods come from "hidden" sugar and fat.

Manufacturers of processed foods are notorious for putting sugar into food that consumers are unaware of. Most people, for example, don't know that Heinz tomato ketchup contains more sugar per volume than Sealtest chocolate ice cream, or that Wishbone Russian dressing contains more sugar per volume than Coca Cola. While Coca Cola is about 9 percent sugar, Wishbone Russian dressing is about 30 percent sugar. Similarly, Coffee-Mate contains 65 percent sugar, more than seven times the amount of sugar per volume of Coca Cola.

Many other foods that are not associated with sweetness are nonetheless high in sugar, and therefore high in calories. To name a very few of them: Dannon lowfat fruit yogurt, 14 percent sugar; Hamburger Helper, 23 percent sugar; Ritz crackers, 12 percent sugar; Shake 'n Bake Barbecue, 51 percent sugar. And what about Jello, the dessert that, according to advertising, there is "always room for"? Jello contains a whopping 83 percent pure sugar!

Sugar does not always add noticeable sweetness, because its taste is often disguised by other foods, such as salt. It is also disguised on the label—as sucrose, glucose, maltose, dextrose, lactose, fructose, dextrins and corn syrup. If you see the suffix "ose," you know you are being fed sugar. Learn to read labels like a hawk, and put back foods with hidden sugar.

Sugar is added to foods because it helps retain moisture, lowers freezing points, preserves food, and seems to provide a taste "addiction" to the foods it is added to. At only about a dime per pound, sugar is a multifaceted bargain for the food processor, but it is no bargain for the consumer. It is a metabolism-disrupting, fattening junk food that the human body has no need for. It does, indeed, as its apologists claim, provide "quick energy," but this quick energy is replaced by an *energy drop* that is *just as quick.*

Every man, woman and child in North America eats an average of 130 pounds of sugar per year, or more than one-third of a pound *each day*. And most of this sugar is hidden in processed foods.

Fat is also found in processed foods, often in the form of shortening or oil. It is also in whole foods not often thought of as high-fat, such as nuts or avocados. A piece of frozen apple pie, for example, which is not an obviously high-fat food, contains about 180 calories of fat! A toaster-heated pop-tart contains about 160 calories of fat. A cup of Brazil nuts contains about 800 calories of fat, and an avocado contains about 210 fat calories. A Salisbury steak TV dinner contains about 480 calories of fat, and six ounces of tuna fish contain about 240 calories of fat. Because an ounce of fat contains about 225 percent more calories than an ounce of sugar, protein or starch, fat calories can add up quickly.

One of the best ways to avoid hidden fat and sugar calories is to avoid processed foods. If a food has been pre-cooked, broken into various components, or mixed with other food products in a package or can, there is a very good chance that it will contain fat or sugar. One of the best pieces of advice that dieters can take is: *"Eat simply."* If dieters were to eat *whole food* products—fresh vegetables and fruits and grains—rather than foods that have been *broken down and boxed and mixed and canned,* they would be on their way to overcoming their weight problems. A good rule of thumb—perhaps overly simplistic but still a good guideline—is: "Eat very little food that comes in a box or a can."

How to Use Our Sample Menu Plans

The menu plans and recipes included in this book are *examples,* not iron-clad rules that must be followed to the letter. A dieter could devise his or her own menu plan without ever using any of our particular meal plans or recipes, if he or she were to simply adhere to the *spirit* of our recommendations.

Because menus for only one week of the weight loss phase and one week of the weight maintenance phase are described in detail in this book, you will, obviously, have to soon devise your own menu plans. You could keep eating our one-week menu plan over and over again, of course, but that would become very boring. You should use our one-week plans as *blueprints,* as examples to pattern your own meal plans after.

The most important rule in planning your meals is to use appropriate amounts of non-starchy foods. As we mentioned in the chapter "How to Use the Starch-Blocker," you should eat 500 non-starch calories, combined with about 700 starch calories, each day during your weight loss phase, and about 700-1,000 starch calories, combined with about 700-1,000 non-starch calories, each day during your weight maintenance phase.

The amount of total calories and starch calories that you eat, and how often you use the starch-blocker, can be adjusted periodically, depending upon the amount of weight you want to lose. You will, of course, lose the most weight if you eat a high-starch, low non-starch diet, and use the starch-blocker frequently. Our maintenance plan recommendations, which call for a maximum processing of 2,400 calories per day—if *no* starch-blocker tablets are used—may not provide sufficient calories for some people, particularly not tall, heavy-set men. If you *continue* to lose unnecessary weight on the maintenance program, *gradually* add more calories until your weight stabilizes at a comfortable level.

To make up your own menu plans, use the calorie tables included in this book. You can write out your menu plans in the blank chart entitled, "My Starch Blocker Menu Plan," or you can create a similar chart of your own.

You can also determine the starch and non-starch caloric contents of your own current favorite recipes by using the starch-content lists in this book. Transcribe these caloric values onto a photocopy or hand-written copy of the blank charts entitled "My Own Favorite Starchy Recipes."

Strive for balance, diversity and taste-appeal in your menu plans. You will stay on this diet only as long as you are content with it, so create meals that you will look forward to.

As we describe in the next chapter, entitled "How to Begin Your Program," you can make detailed meal plans or generalized meal plans, and you can make long-term or short-term plans. You can even delay writing down your menu until after you have eaten, recording it as a food "diary." We recommend that you use relatively detailed long-range planning in the beginning, then shift to less detailed, shorter-range planning as you become accustomed to the starch-blocker weight control program.

This program, because of its supreme effectiveness and the satisfaction it brings dieters, may become the last diet you will ever need—if you apply it correctly.

So plan carefully, keep yourself informed about the caloric contents of the foods you are eating—and get ready to begin the best diet you have ever been on.

Menu Plan: Weight Loss Phase

Sample Menu Plan—Day #1 (weight loss phase)

Food (amount)	Total Calories contained in food	Starch Calories (blocked by starch-blocker)	Non-starch Calories remaining after starch-blocker use
Breakfast			
½ c. fresh strawberries	24	0	24
1 c. rice cereal	85	72	13
¼ c. 2% milk and ½ tsp. sugar	30	0	30
	139	72	67 total calories processed
Snack			
2 saltines	35	32	3 total calories processed
Lunch			
French onion soup with French bread*	240	100	140
lettuce wedge with low-cal dressing	50	0	50
3 vanilla wafers	50	30	20
	340	130	210 total calories processed
Snack			
2 slices of bread with 2 tsp. lite apple butter	225	200	25 total calories processed
Dinner			
Rice and Chicken liver pilau* (small serving)	200	75	125
Cucumber & onion slices (marinated in dill pickle juice) on lettuce leaf	40	0	40
2" square corn bread*	100	80	20
1 c. mashed squash	130	120	10
	470	275	195 total calories processed
TOTAL FOR THE DAY	1,209 total calories eaten during the day	709 total calories blocked by starch-blocker.	500 total calories processed during the day

*indicates recipe included in this book

Sample Menu Plan—Day #2
(weight loss phase)

Food (amount)	Total Calories contained in food	Starch Calories (blocked by starch-blocker)	Non-starch Calories remaining after starch-blocker use
Breakfast			
1 slice banana nut bread	150	34	116
1 plum	30	0	30
	180	34	**146** total calories processed
Snack			
Rye thins	**31**	28	**3** total calories processed
Lunch			
chicken noodle soup	212	160	52
1 biscuit	75	60	15
1 c. skim milk	90	0	90
	377	220	**157** total calories processed
Snack			
1 banana	120	104	**16** total calories processed
Dinner			
Wok chow mein*	251	93	158
1 c. cooked rice	200	180	20
1 ear corn	70	64	6
	521	337	**184** total calories processed
TOTAL FOR THE DAY	1,229 total calories eaten during the day	723 total calories blocked by starch-blocker	506 total calories processed during the day

Sample Menu Plan—Day #3
(weight loss phase)

Food (amount)	Total Calories contained in food	Starch Calories (blocked by starch-blocker)	Non-starch Calories remaining after starch-blocker use
Breakfast			
1 piece French toast*	151	95	56
½ c. milk	45	0	45
1 banana	120	104	16
	316	199	**117** total calories processed
Snack			
1 puffed rice cracker	90	75	**15** total calories processed
Lunch			
1 portion zucchini casserole*	170	67	103
V-8 juice	35	5	30
	205	72	**133** total calories processed
Snack			
2 pieces bread with diet margarine	225	200	**25** total calories processed
Dinner			
1 portion chicken supreme*	245	80	165
1 med. baked potato	120	100	20
	365	180	**185** total calories processed
TOTAL FOR THE DAY	1,201 total calories eaten during the day	726 total calories blocked by starch-blocker	**475** total calories processed during the day

Sample Menu Plan—Day #4
(weight loss phase)

Food (amount)	Total Calories contained in food	Starch Calories (blocked by starch-blocker)	Non-starch Calories remaining after starch-blocker use
Breakfast			
1 poached egg	78	0	78
1 sl. whole wheat toast	110	100	10
½ c. skim milk	45	0	45
	233	100	**133** total calories processed
Snack			
1 banana	120	104	**16** total calories processed
Lunch			
Italian minestrone soup*	207	138	69
¼ small head lettuce wedge with vinaigrette dressing*	20	0	20
2 slices toasted French bread	116	100	16
	343	238	**105** total calories processed
Snack			
4 non-sugared wheat crackers	50	40	10
1 celery stalk	10	0	10
	60	40	**20** total calories processed
Dinner			
1 shrimp stuffed pepper*	215	90	125
½ c. corn pudding*	96	51	45
1 slice bread with 1 tsp. whipped butter	112	100	12
	423	241	**182** total calories processed
TOTAL FOR THE DAY	1,179 total calories eaten during the day	723 total calories blocked by starch-blocker	**456** total calories processed during the day

Sample Menu Plan—Day #5
(weight loss phase)

Food (amount)	Total Calories contained in food	Starch Calories (blocked by starch-blocker)	Non-starch Calories remaining after starch-blocker use
Breakfast			
Cantaloupe (¼ about 5″ in diameter)	30	10	20
Applesauce oatmeal	130	110	20
1 slice bread	110	100	10
	270	220	**50** total calories processed
Snack			
English muffin (½ toasted with 1 tsp. cream cheese	65	45	**20** total calories processed
Lunch			
Macaroni and cheese	290	116	174
Green onions (2)	6	0	6
Radishes (4 small)	5	0	5
No-calorie diet drink	0	0	0
	301	116	**185** total calories processed
Snack			
Rye bread (1 slice toasted)	101	64	37
Beef bouillon (¾ c., hot)	5	0	5
	106	64	**42** total calories processed
Dinner			
Chicken noodle soup	212	160	52
Beef chop suey	310	190	120
Herb tea	0	0	0
	522	350	**172** total calories processed
TOTAL FOR THE DAY	1,264 total calories eaten during the day	795 total calories blocked by starch-blocker	**469** total calories processed during the day

Sample Menu Plan—Day #6
(weight loss phase)

Food (amount)	Total Calories contained in food	Starch Calories (blocked by starch-blocker)	Non-starch Calories remaining after starch-blocker use
Breakfast			
Grapefruit (½ med.)	60	0	60
Rice & raisins (½ c. w/brown sugar (2 tsp.) and cream (2 tsp.)	183	90	93
	243	90	153 total calories processed
Snack			
Toast (1 slice w/1 tsp. whipped butter)	113	100	13
Herb tea	0	0	0
	113	100	13 total calories processed
Lunch			
Meat turnover*	135	68	67
Tossed vegetable salad w/diet dressing	50	0	50
	185	68	117 total calories processed
Snack			
Banana	120	104	16
Skim milk (½ c.)	45	0	45
	165	104	61 total calories processed
Dinner			
Chicken and biscuits*	207	146	61
Baked acorn squash (½ small)	124	110	14
Tomato (1 fresh, sliced)	35	0	35
1 sl. whole wheat bread	108	98	10
	474	354	120 total calories processed
TOTAL FOR THE DAY	1,180 total calories eaten during the day	716 total calories blocked by starch-blocker	464 total calories processed during the day

Sample Menu Plan—Day #7
(weight loss phase)

Food (amount)	Total Calories contained in food	Starch Calories (blocked by starch-blocker)	Non-starch Calories remaining after starch-blocker use
Sunday Brunch			
Scrambled egg (1)	80	0	80
Hash browns & carrots	132	100	32
Toast (1 piece with 1 tsp. whipped butter)	112	100	12
Red raspberries	35	0	35
	359	200	159 total calories processed
Snack			
Rye thins (3)	93	84	9
No-calorie diet drink	0	0	0
	93	84	9 total calories processed
Dinner			
Turkey curry*	375	149	226
Scalloped tomatoes	170	100	70
Banana salad (1 banana sliced onto lettuce leaf topped w/1 T. yogurt & sprinkle of nutmeg)	128	104	24
Bread (1 slice with 1 tsp. whipped butter)	112	100	12
	785	453	332 total calories processed
TOTAL FOR THE DAY	1,237 total calories eaten during the day	737 total calories blocked by starch-blocker	500 total calories processed during the day

Menu Plan: Maintenance Phase

Sample Menu Plan—Day #1 (maintenance phase)

Food (amount)	Total Calories contained in food	Starch Calories (blocked by starch-blocker)	Non-starch Calories remaining after starch-blocker use
Breakfast			
2 eggs	160	0	160
2 pieces toast w/whipped butter	230	200	30
1 banana and 2 T. Half-and-half	160	104	56
Herb tea	0	0	0
	550	304	**246** total calories processed
Snack			
2 sl. toast w/whip butter	230	200	**30** total calories processed
Lunch			
1 chicken sandwich with lo-cal mayonnaise	350	220	130
Cream of potato soup	100	65	35
1 dinner roll	110	100	10
	560	385	**175** total calories processed
Dinner			
3 oz. rump roast, lean	300	0	300
1 dinner salad with vinaigrette dressing	30	0	30
1 baked potato, med.	120	100	20
1 piece bread with whipped butter	120	100	20
1 cup tomato juice	35	0	35
	605	200	**405** total calories processed
Snack			
1 serving corn pudding*	**86**	**51**	**35** total calories processed
TOTAL FOR THE DAY	**2,031** total calories eaten during the day	**1,140** total calories blocked by starch-blocker	**891** total calories processed during the day

*Indicates recipe included in this book

Sample Menu Plan—Day #2
(maintenance phase)

Food (amount)	Total Calories contained in food	Starch Calories (blocked by starch-blocker)	Non-starch Calories remaining after starch-blocker use
Breakfast			
Cold wheat or rice cereal w/1 t. honey	220	80	140
Hot herb tea	0	0	0
1 hot biscuit	75	60	15
1 orange	60	0	60
	355	140	215 total calories processed
Snack			
1 oz. cheese slice	100	0	100
½ apple	40	0	40
	140	0	140 total calories processed
Lunch			
1 serving Easy Chicken and Noodles*	125	80	45
1 c. steamed broccoli	40	0	40
1 piece wh. wheat bread	110	100	10
1 c. tomato juice	35	0	35
	310	180	130 total calories processed
Snack			
2 pieces pumpernickle bread lightly buttered with whipped butter	230	200	30 total calories processed
Dinner			
3 oz. roast turkey, w/o skin, white meat	150	0	150
1 baked sweet potato, medium-sized	180	160	20
1 dinner salad with lo-cal dressing	40	0	40
1 hot dinner roll	100	90	10
1 piece banana cream pie	215	75	140
	685	325	360 total calories processed

Sample Menu Plan—Day #2 (cont.)

Food (amount)	Total Calories contained in food	Starch Calories (blocked by starch-blocker)	Non-starch Calories remaining after starch-blocker use
Snack			
3 c. popcorn	220	180	**40** total calories processed
TOTAL FOR THE DAY	1,940 total calories eaten during the day	1,025 total calories blocked by starch-blocker	**915** total calories processed during the day

Sample Menu Plan—Day #3
(maintenance phase)

Food (amount)	Total Calories contained in food	Starch Calories (blocked by starch-blocker)	Non-starch Calories remaining after starch-blocker use
Breakfast			
4 med. sized pancakes, lightly buttered, with 1 T. honey	420	250	170
1 c. skim milk	90	0	90
½ cantaloupe	80	0	80
Herb Tea or no-calorie drink	0	0	0
	590	250	**340** total calories processed
Snack			
2 pieces rye bread with 1 oz. lo-cal. cream cheese	245	200	**45** total calories processed
Lunch			
3 oz. broiled chicken, without skin	120	0	120
1 ear sweet corn	70	64	6
1 serving Venetian rice and peas*	186	120	66
1 c. V-8 juice	35	0	35
1 dinner salad with lo-cal dressing	40	0	40
	451	184	**267** total calories processed

Sample Menu Plan—Day #3 (cont.)

Food (amount)	Total Calories contained in food	Starch Calories (blocked by starch-blocker)	Non-starch Calories remaining after starch-blocker use
Snack			
2 pieces toasted whole wheat bread w/butter and apple butter	240	200	40 total calories processed
Dinner			
2 c. spaghetti with tomato sauce*	500	296	204
2 pieces garlic bread, lightly buttered	240	200	40
2 oz. white wine	50	0	50
1 dinner salad with lo-cal dressing	40	0	40
	830	496	334 total calories processed
TOTAL FOR THE DAY	2,356 total calories eaten during the day	1,330 total calories blocked by starch-blocker	1,026 total calories processed during the day

Sample Menu Plan—Day #4
(maintenance phase)

Food (amount)	Total Calories contained in food	Starch Calories (blocked by starch-blocker)	Non-starch Calories remaining after starch-blocker use
Breakfast			
2-egg cheese-scallion omelette (with ¼ c. cheddar cheese)	275	0	275
2 biscuits, lightly buttered with whipped butter and apple butter	200	120	80
1 c. hash browns, cooked with non-stick vegetable spray	120	100	20
	595	220	375 total calories processed
Snack			
1 banana and 1 T. Half-and-half	140	104	.36 total calories processed

Sample Menu Plan—Day #4 (cont.)

Food (amount)	Total Calories contained in food	Starch Calories (blocked by starch-blocker)	Non-starch Calories remaining after starch-blocker use
Lunch			
¼ lb. cheeseburger with bun, catsup, mustard, pickle, onion (lean meat)	465	180	285
No-calorie soft drink	1	0	1
Oven-baked french fries (10 pieces)	170	135	35
	636	315	321 total calories processed
Snack			
1 English muffin lightly buttered with whipped butter (both halves)	260	200	60 total calories processed
Dinner			
1 serving broiled fish	80	0	80
1 c. rice with hot curry and mustard sauce*	215	180	35
Lettuce wedge with lo-cal dressing	20	0	20
Herb tea or no-calorie drink	0	0	0
1 c. steamed cauliflower	25	0	25
	340	180	160 total calories processed
Snack			
1 c. beef bouillon	7	0	20
1 piece whole wheat bread, lightly buttered with whipped butter	130	100	30
	150	100	50 total calories processed
TOTAL FOR THE DAY	2,121 total calories eaten during the day	1,119 total calories blocked by starch-blocker	1,002 total calories processed during the day

Sample Menu Plan—Day #5
(maintenance phase)

Food (amount)	Total Calories contained in food	Starch Calories (blocked by starch-blocker)	Non-starch Calories remaining after starch-blocker use
Breakfast			
1 pecan or walnut waffle with lo-cal syrup	250	180	70
Herb tea or no-cal drink	0	0	0
1 sl. beef bacon (extra grease blotted w/napkin)	45	0	45
	295	180	115 total calories processed
Snack			
Raw vegetables dipped in garden sauce*	50	0	50
4 Rye Krisp crackers	124	112	12
	174	112	**62** total calories processed
Lunch			
1 serving broccoli and corn casserole*	115	75	40
1 dinner roll	100	90	10
1 dinner salad with vinaigrette dressing	20	0	20
	235	165	**70** total calories processed
Snack			
1 piece fruit (pear or apple) sliced in wedges	175	0	175
¼ c. cheese	125	0	125
	300	0	**300** total calories processed

Sample Menu Plan—Day #5 (cont.)

Food (amount)	Total Calories contained in food	Starch Calories (blocked by starch-blocker)	Non-starch Calories remaining after starch-blocker use
Dinner			
1 serving macaroni or rigatoni with Spanish sauce* (1½ c. cooked pasta, 1 serving sauce)	357	222	135
1 dinner salad with lo-cal dressing	25	0	25
1 slice garlic bread, lightly buttered with whipped butter	110	100	10
2 oz. white wine	50	0	50
	542	322	220 total calories processed
Snack			
1 c. hard ice milk, with nuts, cinnamon, sliced fresh peaches or other fruit	250	0	250 total calories processed
TOTAL FOR THE DAY	1,796 total calories eaten during the day	779 total calories blocked by starch-blocker	1,017 total calories processed during the day

Sample Menu Plan—Day #6
(maintenance phase)

Food (amount)	Total Calories contained in food	Starch Calories (blocked by starch-blocker)	Non-starch Calories remaining after starch-blocker use
Breakfast			
Fruit salad with vanilla or plain yogurt (1 c. fruit, ½ c. yogurt)	200	0	200
2 pieces toast, lightly buttered with whipped butter and apple butter	240	200	40
Herb tea or no-cal drink	0	0	0
	440	200	240 total calories processed

*indicates recipe included in this book

Sample Menu Plan—Day #6 (cont.)

Food (amount)	Total Calories contained in food	Starch Calories (blocked by starch-blocker)	Non-starch Calories remaining after starch-blocker use
Snack			
8 Rye Krisp	124	112	12
1 c. orange juice	110	0	110
	234	112	**122** total calories processed
Lunch			
1 deep-fried fish sandwich, with mayonnaise	420	200	220
Ice tea with lemon	0	0	0
1 bowl potato soup	100	65	35
	520	265	**255** total calories processed
Snack			
1 banana	120	104	**16** total calories processed
Dinner			
3 slices vegetarian cheese pizza	660	450	210
1 dinner salad with Italian dressing	30	0	30
2 pieces garlic bread, lightly buttered with whipped butter	240	200	40
1 c. tomato juice	35	0	35
1 bowl Italian minestrone soup	207	138	69
	1,172	788	**384** total calories processed
Snack			
1 piece sour cream chocolate cake with cream cheese frosting	275	75	200
Herb tea	0	0	0
	275	75	**200** total calories processed
TOTAL FOR THE DAY	2,761 total calories eaten during the day	1,544 total calories blocked by starch-blocker	**1,217** total calories processed during the day

Sample Menu Plan—Day #7
(maintenance phase)

Food (amount)	Total Calories contained in food	Starch Calories (blocked by starch-blocker)	Non-starch Calories remaining after starch-blocker use
Breakfast			
1 bowl oatmeal, with honey, raisins and milk	200	100	100
1 piece cinnamon toast	125	90	35
1 poached egg	80	0	80
Herb tea or no-cal drink	0	0	0
	405	190	**215** total calories processed
Snack			
1 apple	80	0	80
¼ c. cheese	112	0	112
	192	0	**192** total calories processed
Lunch			
1 chef's salad (with turkey, cheese, egg, assorted vegetables and vinaigrette)	250	0	250
1 dinner roll	110	100	10
1 c. V-8 juice	35	0	35
	395	100	**295** total calories processed
Snack			
1 English muffin (both halves, lightly buttered with whipped butter)	260	200	**60** total calories processed

Sample Menu Plan—Day # 7 (cont.)

Food (amount)	Total Calories contained in food	Starch Calories (blocked by starch-blocker)	Non-starch Calories remaining after starch-blocker use
Dinner			
1 serving cabbage and beef casserole*	152	45	107
1 serving broiled tomato*	45	18	27
1 dinner roll	110	100	10
1 dinner salad with vinaigrette	20	0	20
1 med. baked potato	120	100	20
1 c. fresh frozen peaches	210	0	210
	657	263	394 total calories processed
TOTAL FOR THE DAY	1,909 total calories eaten during the day	753 total calories blocked by starch-blocker	1,156 total calories processed during the day

Starch Content of Foods

Food	Total Calories	Starch Calories (Blocked by Starch-Blocker	Non-Starch Calories Remaining after Starch-Blocker Use
	BREAD		
Flour—1 cup	400	340	60
Bread crumbs—1 cup	330	300	30
Bread—1 slice	110	100	10
Bread croutons—1 cup	220	200	20
Earth Grain Lite Bread —1 slice	110	100	10
Whole wheat bread— 1 slice	108	98	10
Pita bread—1 slice	132	120	12
Pumpernickle bread	114	104	10
"Party" rye bread	45	40	5
Biscuit	75	60	15
Dinner roll	100	90	10
Saltine crackers (4)	70	64	6
Oyster crackers (20)	70	64	6
Rye thins (6)	31	28	3
Rye crisp (2)	31	28	3
Cracker crumbs—1 cup	350	320	30
	CEREALS (All 1 cup measurement)		
Corn meal	380	320	60
Cooked corn meal mush	190	160	30
Corn meal grits	260	235	25
All Bran	200	180	20
Bran Chex	130	120	10
Cheerios	80	65	15
Corn Flakes	100	84	16
Raw barley	760	640	120
Bran Flakes	180	160	20
Hulled oats	500	452	48
Puffed rice	85	72	13
Puffed wheat	65	56	9
Special K	110	70	40
Wheat flakes	110	80	30
Rice, uncooked	600	540	60
Rice, cooked	200	180	20

Food	Total Calories	Starch Calories (Blocked by Starch-Blocker	Non-Starch Calories Remaining after Starch-Blocker Use
PASTA			
(1 lb. dry = 4 cups dry or 8 cups cooked)			
Macaroni—1 cup dry	420	336	84
Macaroni—1 c. cooked	210	168	42
Spaghetti—1 cup raw	420	296	124
Spaghetti—1 c. cooked	210	148	62
Noodles—1 cup raw	350	320	30
Noodles—1 c. cooked	200	183	17
Cheese pizza—1 slice of 10″ pie	212	150	62
VEGETABLES			
(1 lb. raw beans = 2½ cups raw beans or 6 cups cooked)			
Beans, lima or kidney —1 cup raw	528	432	96
Beans, lima or kidney 1 cup cooked	220	180	40
Pinto, navy—1 cup raw	525	450	75
Pinto, navy—1 cup cooked	210	180	30
Corn—1 cup	174	160	14
Corn—1 ear	70	64	6
Rice, cooked—1 cup	200	180	20
Parsnips—1 cup	140	128	12
Peas, canned—1 cup	165	120	45
Potato, baked—small	80	70	10
medium	120	100	20
large	145	120	25
Mashed potato—1 cup	360	300	60
French fries—10 pcs.	170	80	90
Potato chips—10 pcs.	110	40	70
Sweet potato	180	160	20
Sweet potato, canned or mashed—1 cup	280	220	60
Squash, mashed—1 c.	130	120	10
Banana	120	104	16
Tapioca pudding	220	180	40
Tomato spaghetti sauce—1 cup	140	38	102

Quick Reference Calorie Chart

VEGETABLES and JUICES

	Calories
Artichoke, 1 whole	45
Asparagus, canned, 1 cup	45
Asparagus, raw, 1 lb.	66
Beans, green snap, fresh, 1 cup	30
Baked beans, 1 cup	310
Beans, green, frozen, 3½ oz.	25
Beans sprouts, raw, 1 cup	30
Beans, yellow or wax, cooked, 1 cup	22
Beets, canned, 1 cup	85
Beet greens, raw, 1 cup	27
Broccoli, frozen, 1 pkg.	75
Broccoli, raw, 1 lb.	113
Brussel sprouts, raw, 1 lb.	188
Cabbage, green, cooked, 1 cup	30
Cabbage, green, raw, 1 cup (1 small head = 4 cups)	17
Carrot, raw, 1	15
Carrots, cooked, 1 cup	50
Carrots, raw, grated, 1 cup	28
Cauliflower, raw, 1 lb.	122
Cauliflower, cooked, 1 cup	30
Celery, raw, 1 stalk (3 stalks = 1 cup)	7
Chard, raw, 1 lb.	104
Chard, cooked, 1 cup	30
Chicory, raw, 1 cup	10
Chinese cabbage, raw, 1 cup	10
Chinese cabbage, cooked, 1 cup	16
Chives, raw, 1 Tbsp.	4
Collards, raw, 1 lb.	140
Collards, cooked, 1 cup	50
Corn, canned, 1 cup	174
Corn, cream style (canned) 1 cup	210
Corn, cooked on the cob, 1 ear	70
Cress, garden, cooked, 1 cup	30
Cucumber, raw, 1	30

Vegetables and Juices cont.

Dandelion greens, cooked, 1 cup	60
Dandelion greens, raw, 1 lb.	204
Eggplant, cooked, 1 cup	40
Eggplant, raw, 1 lb.	92
Endive, raw, 1 cup	10
Escarole, raw, 1 lb.	47
Garlic, 1 clove	2
Green beans, raw, 1 lb.	128
Green beans, canned, 1 cup	45
Kale, cooked, 1 cup	40
Kale, raw, 1 lb.	130
Kohlrabi, raw, 1 lb.	100
Kohlrabi, cooked, 1 cup	40
Leeks, raw, 1 lb.	123
Lettuce, leaf, 1 leaf	3
Lettuce, iceberg, 1 head	60
Lettuce, shredded & chopped, 1 cup	10
Mushrooms, raw, 1 lb.	127
Mushrooms, canned, 1 cup	40
Mustard greens, raw, 1 lb.	140
Mustard greens, cooked, 1 cup	30
Okra, cooked, cuts & pods, 1 cup	70
Okra, sliced, 1 cup	50
Olive, 1 medium	30
Onion, raw, 1 medium size	40
Onion, green, 1 medium size	8
Onion, chopped, 1 Tbsp.	5
Onion, chopped, 1 cup	80
Onion, cooked, 1 cup	60
Onion rings, fried, 1 oz.	85
Parsnips, cooked, diced, 1 cup	100
Parsnips, mashed, 1 cup	140
Peas, green, canned, 1 cup	165
Peas, green, cooked, 1 cup	145
Pepper, green, 1	16
Pimento, canned, 1	11
Potato, baked, 1 large	145

Vegetables and Juices cont.

Potato, baked, 1 cup	300
Potato, boiled, 1 medium	120
Potato, boiled, 1 small	90
Potato chips, 10	115
Potato, fresh French fried, 10	215
Potato, frozen, heated to serve, 10	170
Potato, pan fried from raw, 1 cup	460
Potato, hash brown, 1 cup	350
Potato, mashed, no milk, 1 cup	120
Potato, mashed, milk added, 1 cup	140
Potato, mashed, milk & fat added, 1 cup	200
Potatoes au gratin, 1 cup	360
Potato, scalloped without cheese, 1 cup	250
Potato salad, with cooked salad dressing, 1 cup	250
Potato salad, with mayonnaise or french dressing & eggs, 1 cup	360
Potato sticks, 1 cup	190
Pumpkin, canned, 1 cup	80
Radishes, raw, 1	1
Rutabagas, cooked, diced, 1 cup	60
Sauerkraut, canned, 1 cup	40
Spinach, raw, 1 lb.	118
Spinach, cooked or canned, 1 cup	50
Squash, summer, raw, 1 lb.	96
Squash, summer, cooked, 1 cup	30
Squash, winter, baked, 1 cup	130
Squash, winter, boiled, 1 cup	90
Sweet potatoes, cooked or baked, 1	160
Sweet potatoes, canned, mashed, 1 cup	280
Sweet potatoes, candied, 1 (8 oz.)	400
Tomatoes, raw, 1 medium	25
Tomatoes, raw, 1 cup, chopped	30
Tomato ketchup, 1 cup	320
Tomatoes, canned, 1 cup	60
Tomato juice, 1 oz.	6
Tomatoes, raw, 1 lb.	90
Tomato sauce, 1 cup	170

Vegetables and Juices cont.

Tomato juice, canned, 1 cup	50
Tomato paste, canned, 1 oz.	23
Turnip, raw (cubed or sliced) 1 cup	40
Turnip, cooked, 1 cup	40
Turnip greens, cooked 1 cup	30
Turnip, raw, 1 lb.	125
Vegetable juice cocktail, 1 cup	40
Water chestnuts, 1	5
Watercress, 1 bunch	20
Yams, raw, 1 lb.	395

COOKED DRIED VEGETABLES

	Calories
Beans, red kidney, 1 lb.	1,320
Beans, raw, 2½ cups	528
Beans, cooked, 6 cups	220
Beans, lima, 1 lb.	1,320
Beans, lima, raw, 1 cup	528
Beans, great northern or navy, 1 lb.	1,050
Beans, great northern or navy, raw, 1 cup	525
Beans, great northern or navy, cooked, 5 cups	210
Pea beans, 1 cup cooked	225
Soy beans, 1 cup cooked	235
Lentils, 1 cup cooked	210
Chick peas, 1 cup cooked	270
Split peas	265

BREADS and CRACKERS

	Calories
Bagel, 1 medium	165
Biscuit, 1 medium	125
Bread, brown, Boston, 1 slice	130
white, 1 slice	110
whole wheat, 1 slice	100
cracked wheat, 1 slice	100
French or Vienna, 1 slice	100
corn, 1 piece	100
raisin, 1 slice	62
date nut, 1 slice	130
crumbs, dry, 1 cup	300
Muffin, corn, 1	120
English, 1	140
blueberry, 1	110
plain, 1	120
Cracker, soda or saltine, 1	17
graham, 1	22
butter, 1	12
cheese, 1	15
rye wafer, 1	20
wheat wafer, 1	10
Crescent rolls, 1	100
Cracker crumbs, 1 cup	300
Flour, white, 1 Tbsp.	25
1 cup	400
¾ cup	300
½ cup	200
¼ cup	100
Flour, whole wheat, 1 Tbsp.	26
1 cup	420
¾ cup	315
½ cup	210
¼ cup	105
Flour, rye, 1 Tbsp.	26
1 cup	420
¾ cup	315

Breads and Crackers cont.

Flour, rye, cont.	
½ cup	210
¼ cup	105
Corn meal, 1 Tbsp.	31
1 cup	502
¾ cup	376
½ cup	251
¼ cup	125

FRUITS

	Calories
Apple, fresh, medium	75
baked, sweetened, medium	190
Apple juice, canned, 1 cup	118
Applesauce, sweetened, 1 cup	220
Applesauce, unsweetened, 1 cup	100
Apple Brown Betty, 1 cup	330
Apricots, fresh, raw, 1 lb.	50
canned, water, 1 cup	85
canned, syrup, 1 cup	210
dried, cooked and unsweetened, 1 cup	220
Avocado, peeled, 1	380
Banana, raw, 1	120
Blackberries, fresh, raw, 1 cup	85
Blueberries, fresh, raw, 1 cup	85
Blueberries, frozen, sweetened, 1 cup	125
Cantaloupe, 1 medium	130
Cherries, raw, 1 cup	80
Cherries, canned, syrup, 1 cup	180
Cranberries, raw, 1 cup	50
Cranberry juice, 1 cup	160
Cranberry sauce, 1 Tbsp.	20
Dates, fresh dried, pitted, 1 cup	500
Figs, dried, 1	50
Figs, canned in syrup, 1 cup	220
Fruit cocktail, canned in syrup, 1 cup	195
Grapefruit, raw, 1	110
Grapefruit, canned, water pack, 1 cup	75
Grapefruit, canned, syrup pack, 1 cup	175
Grapefruit juice, fresh, 1 cup	100
Grapefruit juice, canned, sweetened, 1 cup	130
Gelatin, plain, 1 cup	140
Gelatin, dry, unflavored (35 Tbsp.) 1 cup	560
Gelatin dessert with fruit added, 1 cup	160
Grapes, Concord, etc., 1 cup	65
Grapes, Muscat, Thompson, etc., 1 cup	100

Fruits cont.

Grape juice, 1 cup	165
Guava, 1 medium	60
Honeydew melon, 1 medium slice	132
Lemon, 1 medium	20
Lemon juice, 1 cup	60
Lime, 1	25
Lime juice, 1 cup	80
Mango, 1	150
Nectarine, 1	30
Orange, navel, 1 medium	70
Orange juice, unsweetened, 1 cup	120
Orange juice, fresh, 1 cup	110
Orange marmalade, 1 Tbsp.	55
Papaya, 1	120
Peach, fresh, 1 medium	35
Peaches, canned, water, 1 cup	80
Peaches, canned, syrup, 1 cup	200
Peaches, frozen, sweetened, 1 cup	210
Peaches, dried, cooked, unsweetened, 1 cup	100
Pear, raw, fresh, 1	100
Pears, canned, water, 1 cup	80
Pears, canned, syrup, 1 cup	200
Pineapple, fresh, diced, 1 cup	80
Pineapple, canned, crushed or chunks, 1 cup	190
Pineapple, canned, juice pack, 1 cup	95
Pineapple, canned, water pack, 1 cup	63
Pineapple juice, unsweetened, 1 cup	140
Plantain, 1	155
Plums, raw, 1	25
Plums, canned, 1 cup	200
Pomegranate, 1 medium	60
Prunes, dried, cooked, 1 cup	280
Prunes, dried, sweetened, 1 cup	350
Prune juice, canned, 1 cup	200
Raisins, dried, packed, 1 cup	460
Raspberries, black, fresh, 1 cup	100

Fruits cont.

Raspberries, red, fresh, 1 cup	70
Raspberries, red, frozen, sweetened, 1 cup	225
Raspberries, red, frozen, sweetened, 1 oz.	28
Rhubarb, cooked, sweetened, 1 cup	380
Strawberries, fresh, 1 cup	55
Strawberries, frozen, sweetened, 1 cup	270
Strawberries, frozen, sweetened, 1 oz.	30
Tangerine, 1 medium	40
Tangerine juice, 1 cup	180
Watermelon, 1 4″ x 8″ wedge	110

MILK, CHEESE, EGGS

	Calories
Milk, whole, 1 cup	160
skim, 1 cup	90
2% non-fat, 1 cup	145
condensed, 1 cup	980
evaporated, 1 cup	340
evaporated, skim, 1 cup	170
dried, 1 cup	560
buttermilk, 1 cup	90
Cream, whipping, light, 1 Tbsp.	30
Cream, whipping, heavy, 1 Tbsp.	55
Cream, sour, 1 Tbsp.	25
Cream, whipped, 1 Tbsp.	30
Half-and-half, 1 Tbsp.	20
Imitation whipped topping, 1 Tbsp.	10
Cheese, Cheddar, 1 oz.	115
American processed, 1 oz.	105
American processed, 1 Tbsp.	45
Cheddar, grated, 1 cup	450
1 Tbsp.	28
Blue-Roquefort, 1 oz.	105
Camembert, 1 oz.	85
Cottage, uncreamed, 1 oz.	12
Cheese, Cottage, uncreamed, 1 cup	200
Cottage, creamed (low calorie), 1 oz.	15
1 cup	240
Creamy Cheese, 1 oz.	100
Monterey Jack, 1 oz.	105
Mozarella, 1 oz.	80
shredded, 1 cup	425
1 Tbsp.	26
Parmesan, grated, 1 Tbsp.	20
1 cup	320
Swiss, 1 oz.	105
Yogurt, plain from skim milk, 1 cup	120
Yogurt, plain from whole milk, 1 cup	150

Milk, Cheese, Eggs cont.

Eggs, raw, 1 medium	80
white only, 1	20
yolk only, 1	60
fried, 1	90
omelet, plain, 1	100
poached, 1	80
scrambled, with milk and butter, 1	100

MEAT

	Calories
Beef broth, 1 cup	30
Chuck pot roast, braised, lean only, 1 oz.	55
1 lb. raw w/bone	1,150
lean and fat, 1 oz.	82
Rib roast, lean and fat, 1 oz.	125
lean only, 1 oz.	65
Rump roast, lean and fat, 1 oz.	45
lean only, 1 oz.	45
1 lb. raw	640
Steak, broiled, lean and fat, 1 oz.	110
lean only, 1 oz.	60
round, 1 oz.	75
raw, with bone, 1 lb.	850
sirloin, 1 oz.	80
raw, with bone, 1 lb.	1,240
Hamburger, cooked, lean, 1 oz.	65
raw, 1 lb.	810
cooked, regular, 1 oz.	85
regular, raw, 1 lb.	1,215
Corned beef, canned, 1 oz.	60
Corned beef hash, canned, 1 oz.	50
Beef liver, fried, 1 oz.	70
raw, 1 oz.	40
1 lb.	640
Dried, chipped beef, 1 oz.	57
Dried beef, creamed, 1 cup	400
Lean beef & vegetable stew, homemade, 1 cup	230
Beef tongue, braised, 1 oz.	100
Pork (not recommended)	
Pork chop, fresh, untrimmed, 1 oz.	90
raw, with bone, 1 lb.	1,065
trimmed, 1 oz.	70
Bacon, broiled, 1 slice	45
Canadian, 1 slice	60
Loin roast, lean only, 1 oz.	75
lean and fat, 1 oz.	105

Meat cont.

Ham, cooked, lean only, 1 oz.	60
1 cup (6 oz.)	360
lean and fat, 1 oz.	85
Picnic shoulder, fresh, lean, 1 oz.	70
raw, 1 lb.	1,060
Sausage, links or patty, 1 oz.	125
raw bulk, 1 oz.	65
1 lb.	1,040
Tenderloin, 1 oz.	70
Frankfurter, 1 oz.	85
Chicken	
Broth, 1 cup (7½ oz.)	15
Liver, 1 oz.	47
1 lb.	752
Cooked, no skin, 1 oz.	40
1 cup (3 oz.)	120
Fried, dark meat, no skin, 1 oz.	63
Chicken, fried, dark meat, with skin, 1 oz.	75
light meat, skinned, 1 oz.	55
with skin, 1 oz.	70
breast, skinned, 1 medium	240
drumstick, skinned, 1 medium	100
Roasted, dark, no skin or bone, 1 oz.	50
light, no skin or bone, 1 oz.	47
Chicken pie, 1 lb.	1,000
A la king, 1 oz.	55
Fricassee, 1 oz.	45
Chow mein, 1 oz.	30
Turkey, light meat, no skin, roasted, (1 oz.	50
(1 cup = 3 oz.)	150
dark meat, no skin, roasted, 1 oz.	60
Lamb loin chop, 1 oz.	80
rib chop, 1 oz.	90
roast leg, whole, 1 oz.	70
center cut, 1 oz.	55
liver, raw, 1 oz.	40

Meat cont.

Luncheon meats, bologna, 1 oz.	80
Braunscheweiger, 1 oz.	90
ham, boiled, 1 oz.	65
frankfurter, 1 oz.	90
pork links, cooked, 1 oz.	75
salami, cooked, 1 oz.	90
dry, 1 oz.	130
Vienna sausage, 1 oz.	40

FISH

	Calories
Bass, backed, 1 oz.	70
Bluefish, baked, 1 oz.	45
Clams, raw, meat only, 1 oz.	20
canned with juice, 1 oz.	18
Crab meat, 1 oz.	26
Fish sticks, 1	50
Flounder, 1 oz.	22
Haddock, meat only, 1 oz.	22
Haddock, breaded and fried, 1 oz.	47
Halibut, raw, 1 oz.	28
Lobster, whole, 1 lb.	105
Mackerel, boiled, 1 oz.	60
Ocean perch, raw, 1 oz.	25
breaded and fried, 1 oz.	65
White perch, raw, 1 oz.	12
Oyster, raw, 1 cup	180
Salmon, broiled or baked, 1 oz.	50
canned, pink, 1 oz.	60
red, 1 oz.	70
Sardines, canned in oil, 1 oz.	60
Scallops, 1 oz.	23
Shad, raw, 1 oz.	48
Shrimp, raw, 1 oz. (1 cup = 6 oz.)	30
Trout, raw, 1 oz.	14
Tuna, water pack, canned, 1 oz.	38
1 cup	230
Tuna, oil pack, canned, 1 oz.	75
1 cup = 6½ oz.	488

FATS and OILS, DRESSINGS

	Calories
Butter, regular, 1 T.	100
whipped, 1 T.	65
Cooking fats, vegetable, 1 T.	115
lard, 1 T.	115
1 cup	1,840
salad and cooking oil, 1 T.	120
1 cup	1,920
Salad dressings, blue cheese, 1 T.	75
French, regular, 1 T.	65
French, lo-calorie, 1 T.	15
Italian, 1 T.	85
Italian, lo-calorie, 1 T.	10
Mayonnaise, 1 T.	100
Salad dressing (Kraft, etc.), 1 T.	65
Russian, 1 T.	75
Thousand Island, 1 T.	80
Thousand Island, lo-calorie, 1 T.	25
Margarine, regular, 1 T.	100
whipped, 1 T.	68

NUTS and SEEDS

	Calories
Almonds, shelled, whole, 1 cup	850
pieces, 1 T.	53
Brazil, shelled, whole, 1 cup	900
pieces, 1 T.	60
Cashews, shelled, whole, 1 cup	800
pieces, 1 T.	50
Coconut, grated, 1 cup	800
1 T.	50
Chestnut, water, 1 cup	120
1	5
Peanuts, shelled, roasted, 1 cup	850
1 T.	53
Peanut butter, 1 T.	60
Pecans, shelled, whole, 1 cup	750
chopped, 1 cup	800
1 T.	50
Pine nuts, pignolias, 1 oz.	150
pinion, 1 oz.	180
Pumpkin seeds, shelled, 1 cup	730
1 T.	45
Sesame seeds, hulled, 1 cup	860
1 T.	54
Sunflower seeds, hulled, 1 cup	750
1 T.	45
Walnuts, shelled, whole, 1 cup	650
1 T.	40
chopped, 1 cup	800
1 T.	50

SUGARS, SYRUPS and SWEETS

	Calories
Caramels, 1	36
Chocolate syrup, 1 T.	50
Honey, 1 T.	61
1 cup	975
Molasses, light, 1 T.	50
Maple syrup, 1 T.	60
Sugar, white, 1 T.	45
1 cup	720
¼ cup	180
½ cup	360
¾ cup	540
brown, 1 T.	50
1 cup	800
¼ cup	200
½ cup	400
¾ cup	600
powdered, 1 T.	30
1 cup	480
¼ cup	120

SOUPS

	Calories
beef noodle, 1 cup	70
bouillon, 1 cube	5
chicken gumbo, 1 cup	110
chicken noodle, 1 cup	60
cream of asparagus with water, 1 cup	60
with milk, 1 cup	140
cream of celery with milk, 1 cup	165
cream of mushroom with water, 1 cup	130
with milk, 1 cup	210
split pea, 1 cup	145
oyster with milk, 1 cup	190
tomato with water, 1 cup	90
with milk, 1 cup	170
cream of chicken with water, 1 cup	95
with milk, 1 cup	180
chili sauce, 1 T.	17
chili con carne with beans, canned, 1 cup	335

CEREALS and GRAINS

	Calories
Barley, raw, 1 cup	680
Bran Flakes, 40%, 1 cup	105
with raisins, 1 cup	140
Corn Flakes, 1 cup	98
Corn grits (cooked), 1 cup	126
Corn meal, uncooked, 1 cup	500
Farina, cooked, 1 cup	100
Granola, 1 cup	220
Macaroni (2" pcs.) 1 lb. = 4 cups dry (@420 cup)	1,680
Macaroni (2" pcs.) cooked, 1 cup	210
Macaroni and cheese, baked, 1 cup	470
Noodles, 1 lb. raw (1 lb. raw = 7 cups cooked)	1,400
Noodles, cooked, 1 cup	200
Oats, puffed, 1 cup	100
puffed and sweetened, 1 cup	140
rolled, 1 cup	150
Oatmeal, cooked, 1 cup	130
Rice, white or instant, raw, 1 lb.	1,400
cooked, 1 cup	200
brown, raw, 1 lb.	1,624
cooked, 1 cup	232
puffed, 1 cup	58
wild, 1 lb.	1,130
raw, 1 cup	565
cooked, 1 cup	161
Rice, Spanish, 1 cup	130
Spaghetti, 1 lb. dry (= 6½ cups)	190
Spaghetti with meatballs in tomato sauce	335
Wheat flakes, 1 cup	100
shredded, 1 oz. (1 large biscuit)	95
puffed, 1 cup	55
wheat germ, toasted, 1 cup	400
1 T.	25
cracked or rolled, cooked, 1 cup	180
Flour, white, 1 T.	25

Cereals and Grains cont.

Flour, white, 1 cup	400
¾ cup	300
½ cup	200
¼ cup	100
whole wheat, 1 T.	26
1 cup	420
¾ cup	315
½ cup	210
¼ cup	105
Flour, rye, same as whole wheat	
corn meal, 1 lb.	496
1 T.	31
1 cup	502
¾ cup	376
½ cup	251
¼ cup	125

Rice and Chicken Liver Pilau

(can be cooked in wok)

Total Calories	Starch Calories (Blocked by Starch-Blocker)	Non-starch Calories Remaining After Starch-Blocker Use	Ingredients
630	600	30	1 cup uncooked rice
200	0	200	2 T. margarine
40	0	40	1 medium onion, chopped fine
16	0	16	1 green pepper, chopped fine
752	0	752	16 small chicken livers, halved
0	0	0	salt and pepper
70	0	70	3 T. brandy
1,708	600	1,108	Totals per Recipe
427	200	227	Totals per Large Serving
200	75	125	Totals per Small Serving

Directions: Cook rice until tender. Drain. Heat half the butter in wok or skillet, add onions and green pepper and saute for about 5 minutes. Push vegetables to one side and cook half the chicken livers until nicely browned on all sides and done through. Combine vegetables-liver mixture with the cooked rice, season with salt and pepper to taste and keep warm while you heat the remaining butter in a saucepan or wok and cook remaining chicken livers. Heat brandy, ignite with a match, spoon over chicken livers. Keep basting them with the flaming juice until the flame dies. Place rice mixture around edge of serving platter and spoon the brandied chicken livers into the center. Garnish with sprigs of parsley. Serves 4-8.

PLEASE NOTE THAT ALL RECIPE INGREDIENTS HAVE NON-STARCH AND STARCH CALORIES DESIGNATED, SO THAT IF YOU ALTER RECIPES, YOU WILL STILL KNOW CALORIC AMOUNTS.

Garden Sauce
(for rice or pasta)

Total Calories	Starch Calories (Blocked by Starch-Blocker)	Non-starch Calories Remaining After Starch-Blocker Use	Ingredients
30	0	30	1 large cucumber, peeled and seeded
30	0	30	1 small onion, chopped
0	0	0	1 T. parsley
0	0	0	¼ c. juice from Kosher dill pickles
0	0	0	½ tsp. salt
60	0	60	Totals per Recipe
30	0	30	Totals per Serving

Directions: Blend in blender until smooth. Serve with hot rice or pasta which has been tossed with a touch of Parmesan and butter-flavored salt. Serves 2.

Zucchini Casserole

Total Calories	Starch Calories (Blocked by Starch-Blocker)	Non-starch Calories Remaining After Starch-Blocker Use	Ingredients
400	0	400	4 med. zucchini, sliced ½″ thick
30	0	30	1 c. carrots, sliced
40	0	40	1 onion, chopped
440	400	40	2 c. herb-flavored stuffing cubes
95	0	95	1 can cream of chicken soup
15	0	15	½ c. chicken bouillon
1,020	400	620	Totals per Recipe
170	67	103	Totals per Serving

Directions: Cook zucchini, carrots, and onion until just tender. Drain and mix with the stuffing cubes, soup and bouillon. Put in buttered casserole and bake at 350° about 30 minutes. Makes 6-7 servings.

Spanish Sauce
(for rice or pasta)

Total Calories	Starch Calories (Blocked by Starch-Blocker)	Non-starch Calories Remaining After Starch-Blocker Use	Ingredients
0	0	0	1 T. green salsa jalapena or 2 canned green chilies
60	0	60	1 c. lemon juice
30	0	30	1 small onion, chopped
0	0	0	1 clove garlic, diced
25	0	25	1 tomato, peeled and seeded
0	0	0	½ tsp. salt
115	0	115	Totals per Recipe
29	0	29	Totals per Serving

Directions: Place all in blender until smooth. Serve heated. Serves 4.

Wok Sauce

Total Calories	Starch Calories (Blocked by Starch-Blocker)	Non-starch Calories Remaining After Starch-Blocker Use	Ingredients
16	0	16	1 green pepper, chopped fine
7	0	7	1 stalk of celery, sliced thin
30	0	30	1 c. sprouts
30	0	30	1 small onion, sliced and divided into rings
15	0	15	1 carrot, sliced very thin
50	0	50	2 tomatoes, drained, seeded, chopped
200	0	200	½ c. cooking wine
0	0	0	½ tsp. salt
120	0	120	1 T. oil for wok
468	0	468	Totals per Recipe
117	0	117	Totals per Serving

Directions: Prepare all of the vegetables. Heat oil in wok, then stir fry vegetables, starting with carrots and green pepper. When vegetables are done, add the salt and cooking wine. Serves 4 (½ cup slivered almonds sprinkled on top are nice for those on maintenance diet.) Serve with rice or pasta.

Tuna Cakes

Total Calories	Starch Calories (Blocked by Starch-Blocker)	Non-starch Calories Remaining After Starch-Blocker Use	Ingredients
247	0	247	1 6 ½-oz. can water-packed tuna
50	0	50	1 c. cooked, chopped spinach
10	0	10	1 T. minced onion
80	0	80	1 egg
70	64	6	12 soda crackers, crumbled
457	64	393	Totals per Recipe
114	16	98	Totals per Serving

Directions: Place all ingredients in a bowl and mix well. Melt 1 T. vegetable oil in non-stick skillet. Shape tuna mixture into four cakes and brown slowly in hot fat. Serves 4.

Double-baked Potatoes

Total Calories	Starch Calories (Blocked by Starch-Blocker)	Non-starch Calories Remaining After Starch-Blocker Use	Ingredients
480	400	80	4 med. baking potatoes
45	0	45	½ c. skim milk
20	0	20	2 T. yogurt
0	0	0	butter-flavored salt, pepper to taste
0	0	0	1 T. chopped chives
545	400	145	Totals per Recipe
136	100	36	Totals per Serving

Directions: Bake scrubbed potatoes in oven or microwave until soft. Cool to where they can be handled comfortably. Slice in half and scoop centers into bowl. Add other ingredients and beat until light and fluffy. Mound the whipped potato into the shells and return to oven until thoroughly heated through. Serves 4.

Wok Chow Mein

Total Calories	Starch Calories (Blocked by Starch-Blocker)	Non-starch Calories Remaining After Starch-Blocker Use	Ingredients
800	720	80	4 c. cooked rice
880	0	880	1 lb. white chicken meat, sliced into thin strips
40	0	40	1 onion, sliced
20	0	20	1 c. celery, sliced
10	0	10	½ c. bamboo shoots, drained
8	0	8	½ green pepper, diced
25	0	25	1 tomato, chopped
120	0	120	1 small can water chestnuts, drained and sliced
30	0	30	1 c. bean sprouts
60	0	60	1 c. snow pea pods
40	0	40	1 c. mushrooms, sliced
0	0	0	¼ tsp. minced ginger root
30	25	5	1 T. cornstarch
0	0	0	1 c. water
16	0	16	2 T. soy sauce
2,079	745	1,334	Totals per Recipe
259	93	167	Totals per Serving

Directions: Spray wok with no-stick vegetable spray and add chicken and sliced onion; cook two minutes, stirring. Add celery, pepper, and ginger. Cook 2 minutes, stirring. Add water chestnuts, bean sprouts, pea pods, mushrooms, and tomato and cook and stir 2 more minutes. Mix cornstarch with water. Add to vegetables with soy sauce. Simmer for about 10 minutes. Season to taste and serve over hot rice. Serves 8.

Broiled Tomato

Total Calories	Starch Calories (Blocked by Starch-Blocker)	Non-starch Calories Remaining After Starch-Blocker Use	Ingredients
25	0	25	1 tomato
0	0	0	1 T. chopped parsley
20	18	2	1 T. bread crumbs
0	0	0	1 tsp. chopped chives
0	0	0	salt & pepper to taste
45	18	27	Totals per Recipe/Serving

Directions: Cut tomato in half. Sprinkle each half with the spices and herbs, and top with the crumbs. Broil for about 10 minutes.

Barley Soup

Total Calories	Starch Calories (Blocked by Starch-Blocker)	Non-starch Calories Remaining After Starch-Blocker Use	Ingredients
115	0	115	1 T. oil
15	0	15	3 T. onions, chopped
380	320	60	½ c. barley
120	0	120	4 c. hot broth
120	0	120	2 egg yolks, well beaten
160	0	160	1 c. milk
0	0	0	2 T. parsley, finely chopped
910	320	590	Totals per Recipe
228	80	148	Totals per Serving

Directions: Saute onions in oil till clear. Add barley and stir to coat the barley well with oil. Cook 5 minutes. Add broth. Cover and cook 30 minutes or until barley is tender. Remove from heat and stir in eggs and milk. Heat, but do not boil. Sprinkle with chopped parsley. Serves 4.

Sunshine Sauce
(Fruit sauce for rice, especially good served with fish or poultry)

Total Calories	Starch Calories (Blocked by Starch-Blocker)	Non-starch Calories Remaining After Starch-Blocker Use	Ingredients
110	0	110	1 c. orange juice
50	0	50	1 fresh orange, peeled and separated into wedges
55	0	55	1 T. orange marmalade
0	0	0	1 T. cornstarch
215	0	215	Totals per Recipe
56	0	56	Totals per Serving

Directions: Heat orange juice and marmalade in small sauce pan and thicken with the tablespoon of cornstarch which you mix with about 2 tablespoons of water to make a paste before stirring it into the orange juice. Cook and stir until thickened and clear. Remove from heat and add the orange wedges. Spoon over rice. Serves 4.

Popeye Sauce
(for rice and pasta)

Total Calories	Starch Calories (Blocked by Starch-Blocker)	Non-starch Calories Remaining After Starch-Blocker Use	Ingredients
118	0	118	1 pkg. frozen, chopped spinach (or cleaned, cooked and chopped fresh spinach)
60	0	60	½ c. low-fat yogurt
0	0	0	1 tsp. soy sauce
45	0	45	1 T. toasted sunflower seeds
223	0	223	Totals per Recipe
56	0	56	Totals per Serving

Directions: Blend chopped spinach (thawed and drained if you use the frozen, or just drained well if you cook your own), yogurt and soy sauce in blender. Taste. It may need a touch more salt. If so, celery salt goes well. Add the sunflower seeds. Heat and serve. Serves 4.

Cabbage and Beef Casserole

Total Calories	Starch Calories (Blocked by Starch-Blocker)	Non-starch Calories Remaining After Starch-Blocker Use	Ingredients
68	0	68	1 small head of cabbage
20	0	20	½ c. chopped onion
405	0	405	¼ lb. lean ground round
300	270	30	½ c. uncooked rice
120	0	120	2 c. cooked tomatoes
0	0	0	1 c. hot water
0	0	0	1 tsp. salt
0	0	0	½ tsp. pepper
913	270	643	Totals per Recipe
152	45	107	Totals per Serving

Directions: Cut cabbage into 6 wedges and arrange cut-sides up in buttered casserole. Mix the onion, ground round and rice. Place this between the cabbage wedges. Mix seasonings, water and tomatoes and pour over the other ingredients. Cover and bake at 350° for about 1½ hours. Serves 6.

Scalloped Tomatoes

Total Calories	Starch Calories (Blocked by Starch-Blocker)	Non-starch Calories Remaining After Starch-Blocker Use	Ingredients
150	0	150	6 med. tomatoes, peeled
40	0	40	1 med. onion, diced
7	0	7	1 stalk celery, diced
440	400	40	4 slices whole wheat bread, toasted and cubed to 1"
0	0	0	1 tsp. salt
0	0	0	½ tsp. pepper
45	0	45	1 T. sugar
682	400	282	Totals per Recipe
170	100	70	Totals per Serving

Directions: Butter baking dish which has a cover. Slice three of the tomatoes into the baking dish and sprinkle with half of the onion, celery, bread cubes, salt, pepper and sugar. Repeat. Cover dish and bake in moderate oven about 30 minutes. Remove cover and contiue baking until top is crisped. Serves 4.

French Toast

Total Calories	Starch Calories (Blocked by Starch-Blocker)	Non-starch Calories Remaining After Starch-Blocker Use	Ingredients
80	0	80	1 egg
22	0	22	¼ c. milk
0	0	0	½ tsp. vanilla
200	190	10	2 slices bread
302	190	112	Totals per Recipe
151	95	56	Totals per Serving

Directions: Beat together egg, milk and vanilla. Dip bread slices into the mixture and cook in butter melted in skillet until brown on both sides. Serve with low-cal syrup or applesauce. Serves 2.

Hot Curry and Mustard Sauce
(for rice and pasta)

Total Calories	Starch Calories (Blocked by Starch-Blocker)	Non-starch Calories Remaining After Starch-Blocker Use	Ingredients
60	0	60	2 c. chicken broth
25	25	0	1 T. cornstarch
0	0	0	1 T. curry powder
0	0	0	1 tsp. dry mustard
0	0	0	1 T. caraway seed
85	25	60	Totals per Recipe
21	6	15	Totals per Serving

Directions: Make paste of the cornstarch and ¼ cup chicken broth. Heat the remainder of the broth, stir in the cornstarch paste and cook and stir till thickened and clear. Add curry powder, dry mustard and caraway seed. This is best made several hours ahead of time, then reheated just before serving. This allows the spices to blend and reach their peak of tastiness. Just be sure you keep it covered during the waiting period so skin won't form on top. If skin does form, remove it before reheating. Serves 4.

French Onion Soup

Total Calories	Starch Calories (Blocked by Starch-Blocker)	Non-starch Calories Remaining After Starch-Blocker Use	Ingredients
200	0	200	4 large onions, sliced thin
120	0	120	1 T. sesame oil
180	0	180	6 c. beef broth or bouillon
2	0	2	1 tsp. Worcestershire sauce
440	400	40	8 slices from small French loaf or hard rolls
20	0	20	1 T. Parmesan cheese
962	400	562	Totals per Recipe
240	100	140	Totals per Serving

Directions: Cook onions in oil until tender and golden. Add broth and Worcestershire. Cover and simmer 20 minutes. Season with salt and pepper. Pour soup in ovenproof bowls. Float toast slice on top. Sprinkle toast with Parmesan cheese. Slip under broiler till cheese melts (about 4 minutes). Serves 4.

Broccoli and Corn Casserole

Total Calories	Starch Calories (Blocked by Starch-Blocker)	Non-starch Calories Remaining After Starch-Blocker Use	Ingredients
75	0	75	2 c. fresh or 1 pkg frozen broccoli
348	320	28	1 can cream style corn
0	0	0	1 tsp. minced onion
160	0	160	2 eggs, beaten
330	300	30	1 c. cracker crumbs
0	0	0	salt and pepper
913	620	293	Totals per Recipe
114	77	37	Totals per Serving

Directions: Combine all ingredients, except for about ¼ cup of the cracker crumbs. Pour the mixture into a buttered casserole and top it with the reserved crumbs. Bake in a pre-heated 375° oven for about 50 minutes, or until the broccoli is tender. Serves 8.

Parsnip Souffle

Total Calories	Starch Calories (Blocked by Starch-Blocker)	Non-starch Calories Remaining After Starch-Blocker Use	Ingredients
280	256	24	2 c. cooked mashed parsnips (approx. 6)
720	600	120	2 c. mashed potatoes (seasoned with milk, butter, salt and pepper)
160	0	160	2 eggs, yolks separated from whites
25	20	5	1 T. flour
1,185	876	309	Totals per Recipe
296	219	77	Totals per Serving for 4
198	146	52	Totals per Serving for 6

Directions: Peel parsnips and cook until tender in boiling, salted water. Drain. Remove woody vein down center and mash remaining parsnips with potato masher or use blender. Combine mashed parsnips, potatoes, egg yolks and flour. Beat egg whites until fluffy but not dry. Blend carefully into vegetable mixture and spoon mixture into well-buttered casserole. Place in 350° oven and bake about 30 minutes. Serves 4-6.

Chicken and Biscuits

Total Calories	Starch Calories (Blocked by Starch-Blocker)	Non-starch Calories Remaining After Starch-Blocker Use	Ingredients
240	0	240	2 c. cooked chicken, cubed
60	0	60	2 c. chicken broth
600	540	60	2 c. potatoes, cubed
15	0	15	1 c. carrots sliced
40	0	40	1 onion, diced
10	0	10	2 stalks celery, sliced
90	90	0	3 T. cornstarch
0	0	0	salt and pepper
600	540	60	1 tube refrigerator biscuits
1,655	1,170	485	Totals per Recipe
207	146	61	Totals per Serving

Directions: Bring broth to a boil and add potatoes, carrots, onion and celery. Cook until vegetables are tender. Make a paste of cornstarch and thicken the broth. Add chicken. Season, and pour into large casserole or baking dish. While still hot, top with the biscuits and place in oven that has been preheated to 400°. Bake until biscuits are well browned and cooked through. Serves 8.

Pineapple and Banana Sauce for Rice

Total Calories	Starch Calories (Blocked by Starch-Blocker)	Non-starch Calories Remaining After Starch-Blocker Use	Ingredients
190	0	190	1 c. crushed pineapple with juice
240	208	32	2 medium bananas
0	0	0	½ tsp. nutmeg
0	0	0	½ T. cornstarch
45	0	45	1 T. sugar
475	208	267	Totals per Recipe
118	52	66	Totals per Serving

Directions: Drain juice from crushed pineapple and add enough water to it to make one cup. Make a paste of the cornstarch, sugar and two tablespoons of the juice. Use this to thicken the remainder of the juice which you have heated in a small saucepan. When thickened and clear, add nutmeg. Chill in refrigerator. Just before serving, slice or cube the two bananas into the sauce and serve over rice. Serves 4.

Chicken Supreme

Total Calories	Starch Calories (Blocked by Starch-Blocker)	Non-starch Calories Remaining After Starch-Blocker Use	Ingredients
480	0	480	2 chicken breasts
315	300	15	½ c. raw long-grain rice
10	0	10	½ c. chopped celery
20	0	20	2 green onions, diced
30	0	30	1 c. alfalfa or bean sprouts
30	0	30	1 can chicken broth
70	0	70	1 fresh orange
25	20	5	1 T. flour
980	320	660	Totals per Recipe
245	80	165	Totals per Serving

Directions: Cook rice till tender. While rice cooks, remove meat from chicken breasts so you have four pieces (one from each side of the breast). Pound the chicken breast fillets slightly to flatten to about ½-inch thickness. Make a gravy by using enough of the chicken broth to make a paste of the flour, then add this paste to the remaining broth when it is brought to a boil in a small saucepan. Add the chopped celery and onions, and the sprouts to the rice and pour this mixture into a casserole. Top with the chicken fillets. Peel and slice the orange and place the slices about the top of the casserole. Pour the thickened broth over all. Cover and bake at 375° for about 30 minutes. Uncover and bake ten minutes more. Serves four.

Scalloped Zucchini

Total Calories	Starch Calories (Blocked by Starch-Blocker)	Non-starch Calories Remaining After Starch-Blocker Use	Ingredients
260	240	20	2 c. zucchini, sliced ⅛" thick
660	600	60	2 c. bread crumbs
30	30	30	1 c. chicken broth
0	0	0	salt and pepper to taste
950	840	110	Totals per Recipe
158	140	18	Totals per Serving

Directions: Butter casserole. Make a layer of half the zucchini and bread crumbs. Repeat. Pour the broth and sprinkle top crumbs with grated cheese. Cover and bake 30 minutes at 350°. Uncover and bake until crumbs are brown. Serves 6.

Oven Baked French Fries

Total Calories	Starch Calories (Blocked by Starch-Blocker)	Non-starch Calories Remaining After Starch-Blocker Use	Ingredients
480	400	80	4 baking potatoes, med.
173	0	170	1½ T. cooking oil
653	400	253	Totals per Recipe
163	100	63	Totals per Serving

Directions: Potatoes may be pared, or, if you like to eat the peelings, simply scrub well. Slice each potato into 10 french-fry slices. Use pastry brush or the palms of your hands to oil each of the potato slices. Spread them on a non-stick cookie sheet or other pan large enough to allow a space around each "fry." Bake in preheated 400°-450° oven until top and sides are browned, then turn so bottom of the slice is exposed and continue baking until that, too, is brown. Sprinkle with butter-flavored salt and serve hot. Makes 4 servings of 10 french fries for each serving.

Angel Food Cake

Total Calories	Starch Calories (Blocked by Starch-Blocker)	Non-starch Calories Remaining After Starch-Blocker Use	Ingredients
400	340	60	1 c. sifted cake flour
720	0	720	1½ c. sifted confectioners sugar
240	0	240	1½ c. egg whites (about 12)
0	0	0	1½ tsp. cream of tartar
0	0	0	¼ tsp. salt
0	0	0	1 tsp. vanilla
720	0	720	1 c. granulated sugar
2,080	340	1,740	Totals per Recipe
208	34	174	Totals per Serving

Directions: Sift the flour with confectioners sugar two or three times. Beat the egg whites with the cream of tartar, salt and vanilla until stiff enough to make soft peaks but still shiny. Beat in the granulated sugar, 2 T. at a time, and continue beating until the meringue holds stiff peaks. Sift about ¼ of the flour mixture over the whites. Fold in with circular motions and continue until all flour is added. Bake in ungreased 10-inch tube pan in moderate oven (375°) for 30 minutes or until an inserted toothpick comes out clean. Invert pan and cool before removing to cake plate. Serves 10.

Apple Brown Betty

Total Calories	Starch Calories (Blocked by Starch-Blocker)	Non-starch Calories Remaining After Starch-Blocker Use	Ingredients
240	0	240	⅓ c. sugar
0	0	0	½ tsp. each cinnamon & nutmeg
0	0	0	1 T. lemon juice
420	400	20	2 c. bread cubes
900	0	900	3 c. apples, sliced
1,560	400	1,160	Totals per Recipe
290	67	223	Totals per Serving

Directions: In a buttered casserole, alternate layers of apples and bread cubes, and sprinkle each layer with the sugar, cinnamon, nutmeg and lemon juice. Cover and bake at 375° for about 40 minutes. Remove cover and bake about 10 more minutes to brown top crumb layer. Serves 6.

Bean Town Beans

Total Calories	Starch Calories (Blocked by Starch-Blocker)	Non-starch Calories Remaining After Starch-Blocker Use	Ingredients
1,575	1,350	225	3 c. pea or navy beans
270	0	270	6 slices bacon (optional)
0	0	0	1 T. dry mustard
0	0	0	1 tsp. each salt & pepper
400	0	400	½ c. molasses
30	0	30	1 small onion, diced
25	0	25	1 tomato, chopped
15	0	15	1 carrot, diced
2,315	1,350	965	Totals per Recipe
386	225	161	Totals per Serving

Directions: Clean beans. Cover with cold water and soak overnight. Next day, drain, cover with fresh water and boil slowly until tender. Drain, mix in remainder of ingredients and put in bean pot, adding enough boiling water to come to top of beans. Cover pot and bake in slow oven (250°-300°) for about 4 hours. Check from time to time to see if water is needed to keep beans from being too dry. These can also be cooked according to directions for cooking in your favorite crock pot or slow cooker. Serves 6. Great with cornbread and cole slaw.

Scalloped Potatoes . . . with variations

Total Calories	Starch Calories (Blocked by Starch-Blocker)	Non-starch Calories Remaining After Starch-Blocker Use	Ingredients
720	600	120	6 med. potatoes, sliced very thin
180	0	180	2 c. skim milk
50	48	2	2 T. flour
0	0	0	butter-flavored salt and pepper to taste
950	648	302	Totals per Recipe
238	162	76	Totals per Serving

Directions: Use ¼ cup of the milk to mix with flour. Heat remainder of the milk to boiling and thicken with the flour thickener. Season with butter-flavored salt and pepper. Place the sliced potatoes in a buttered casserole and pour the white sauce over them. Bake covered for 45 minutes in a 375° oven. Uncover and bake about 10 more minutes. Serves 4.

Variations: Sliced onions, carrots, or celery (or all three) may be layered into this casserole along with the potatoes.

Venetian Rice and Peas

Total Calories	Starch Calories (Blocked by Starch-Blocker)	Non-starch Calories Remaining After Starch-Blocker Use	Ingredients
600	540	60	1 c. uncooked white rice
90	0	90	2 slices bacon, diced
40	0	40	1 onion, minced
247	180	67	1 pkg. frozen peas or 1½ c. fresh
60	0	60	2 c. chicken broth
80	0	80	¼ c. grated Parmesan cheese
1,117	720	397	Totals per Recipe
186	120	66	Totals per Serving

Directions: Saute bacon in large skillet until crisp. Remove bacon and drain fat from skillet before using it to stir fry onion and peas for about 5 minutes. Add rice to vegetables and continue stirring until rice is lightly browned. Add broth, and salt and pepper to taste. Cover and simmer for about 30 minutes, or until rice absorbs all of the liquid and is tender. Add cheese and crisp, crumbled bacon bits. Makes a nice lunch when served with a salad. Serves 6.

Dutch Cabbage Rolls

Total Calories	Starch Calories (Blocked by Starch-Blocker)	Non-starch Calories Remaining After Starch-Blocker Use	Ingredients
405	0	405	½ lb. lean, ground round steak
300	270	30	½ c. uncooked white rice
40	0	40	1 onion, chopped fine
340	30	310	1 can tomato sauce
10	0	10	½ c. celery, chopped
0	0	0	1 tsp. minced parsley
20	0	20	½ c. mushrooms, sliced
10	0	10	6 large cabbage leaves
1,125	300	825	Totals per Recipe
188	50	138	Totals per Serving

Directions: Cook rice in lightly salted water approximately ½ hour or until done. Remove 6 nice, large leaves from head of cabbage. Slice off top of the big center vein to make leaves more pliable. Drop the cabbage leaves into boiling, salted water for about two minutes. Drain and set aside to dry while you brown the ground beef to which you have added the onion, celery, and mushrooms. Drain fat from the meat mixture and mix the meat with the rice. Place about ½ cup of the rice and meat in the middle of each cabbage leaf. Fold the cabbage leaves around the meat and secure with toothpicks. Place the cabbage rolls in a casserole. Add parsley, salt and pepper to the tomato sauce and pour this over the rolls. Cover and bake at 350° for about 50 minutes. Uncover and bake 15 minutes more. Serves 6.

Easy Chicken and Noodles

Total Calories	Starch Calories (Blocked by Starch-Blocker)	Non-starch Calories Remaining After Starch-Blocker Use	Ingredients
240	0	240	2 c. cubed, cooked chicken
60	0	60	1 qt. chicken broth
0	0	0	salt and pepper
700	640	60	1 pkg. or 2 c. homemade noodles
1,000	640	360	Totals per Recipe
125	80	40	Totals per Serving

Directions: Bring broth to boil. Add noodles and simmer until they are tender. Add chicken and seasonings. If broth is too thin, thicken with 1 T. flour mixed with ¼ c. water. Serves 8.

Hashed Browned Potatoes and Carrots

Total Calories	Starch Calories (Blocked by Starch-Blocker)	Non-starch Calories Remaining After Starch-Blocker Use	Ingredients
720	600	120	6 potatoes, grated
30	0	30	2 large carrots, grated
40	0	40	1 onion, minced
0	0	0	1 tsp. celery salt and pepper to taste
790	600	190	Totals per Recipe
132	100	32	Totals per Serving

Directions: Mix all ingredients. Heat 2 T. cooking oil in non-stick frying pan. Add vegetables and cook slowly until well browned on bottom. Fold as for omelet. Turn heat as low as possible, add 1 T. water, cover skillet and let steam for about 10 minutes or until vegetables are tender in center. Then remove cover to crisp bottom of potatoes again. This also works well if you remove potatoes from skillet after the bottom is well browned and place them on a container suitable for microwave oven use. This way you simply place the browned potatoes in the microwave to finish cooking through. Serves 6.

Corn Pudding

Total Calories	Starch Calories (Blocked by Starch-Blocker)	Non-starch Calories Remaining After Starch-Blocker Use	Ingredients
348	320	28	1 can cream style corn
160	0	160	2 eggs
90	0	90	1 c. skim milk
70	64	6	12 soda crackers, rolled or crumbled
25	24	1	1 T. flour
0	0	0	½ tsp. baking powder
0	0	0	butter-flavored salt and pepper to taste
693	408	285	Totals per Recipe
116	69	47	Totals per Serving

Directions: Separate the eggs and beat whites until stiff. Mix all other ingredients together and fold in beaten egg whites. Pour into buttered casserole and bake at 375° for about 1 hour. Serves 6.

Macaroni and Cheese

Total Calories	Starch Calories (Blocked by Starch-Blocker)	Non-starch Calories Remaining After Starch-Blocker Use	Ingredients
840	672	168	1 8-oz. pkg. elbow macaroni
450	0	450	1 c. Cheddar cheese, grated
180	0	180	2 c. skim milk
25	24	1	1 T. flour
70	0	70	1 T. whipped butter
0	0	0	salt and pepper
1,565	696	869	Totals per Recipe
261	116	145	Totals per Serving

Directions: Cook macaroni in salted water until just tender. Make white sauce by melting the butter, stirring in the flour, and slowly adding milk, and cooking until thickened. Season the sauce with butter-flavored salt and pepper, and add ¾ cup of the grated cheese, plus the macaroni. Place in a buttered baking dish. Sprinkle remainder of the cheese on top. Bake in moderate (375°) oven for about 50-60 minutes. Serves 6.

Vinaigrette Salad Dressing

Total Calories	Starch Calories (Blocked by Starch-Blocker)	Non-starch Calories Remaining After Starch-Blocker Use	Ingredients
8	0	8	½ c. red wine vinegar
6	0	6	2 tsp. onion, grated
0	0	0	2 tsp. parsley, chopped
4	0	4	1 T. dill pickle, chopped
0	0	0	1 T. water
0	0	0	½ tsp. coarse black pepper
0	0	0	1 clove garlic (optional)
0	0	0	1 tsp. celery salt
18	0	18	Totals per Recipe
9	0	9	Totals per Serving

Directions: Place all ingredients in blender. Mix and serve immediately or keep refrigerated in covered jar. Makes 2 servings.

Italian Minestrone

Total Calories	Starch Calories (Blocked by Starch-Blocker)	Non-starch Calories Remaining After Starch-Blocker Use	Ingredients
60	0	60	1 c. tomatoes, chopped
420	360	60	2 c. cooked navy or pea beans
40	0	40	1 large onion, chopped
45	0	45	3 carrots, diced
20	0	20	3 stalks diced celery, leaves & all
17	0	17	1 c. finely shredded cabbage
360	300	60	1 c. raw potatoes, diced
0	0	0	1 clove garlic, minced
210	168	42	1 c. cooked macaroni
60	0	60	2 c. beef broth
0	0	0	3 c. water
1,232	828	404	Totals per Recipe
205	138	67	Totals per Serving

Directions: Bring water to boil and add all of the ingredients except the cooked beans and macaroni. Salt and simmer about 30 minutes. Add broth, beans and macaroni and simmer 10 minutes. Serve topped with parsley sprigs. Serves 6.

Scalloped Chicken

Total Calories	Starch Calories (Blocked by Starch-Blocker)	Non-starch Calories Remaining After Starch-Blocker Use	Ingredients
735	588	147	1 pkg. Creamettes, uncooked
260	0	260	2 cans mushroom soup
30	0	30	2 c. chicken broth
160	0	160	2 hard cooked eggs
460	0	460	¼ lb. cheese, cubed
240	0	240	2 c. chicken, cooked and cubed
1,885	588	1,297	Totals per Recipe
236	74	162	Totals per Serving

Directions: Mix all ingredients in large casserole. Let stand in refrigerator overnight, or for 12 hours. Top with bread crumbs. Bake one hour in moderate oven. Serves 8.

Turkey Curry

Total Calories	Starch Calories (Blocked by Starch-Blocker)	Non-starch Calories Remaining After Starch-Blocker Use	Ingredients
300	0	300	2 c. cooked turkey, diced
0	0	0	1 T. curry powder
70	0	70	1 T. whipped butter
40	0	40	1 onion, minced
20	0	20	1 c. celery, diced
300	0	300	1 c. apple, diced
20	0	20	½ c. sliced mushrooms
60	0	60	2 c. chicken broth
60	56	4	2 T. cornstarch
0	0	0	salt and pepper
600	540	60	3 c. hot cooked rice
1,470	596	874	Totals per Recipe
368	149	219	Totals per Serving

Directions: Melt butter, add curry powder, and stir till browned. Add vegetables and apple. Mix. Add chicken broth and bring to a boil. Combine cornstarch with enough water to make paste and use this to thicken the curry mixture. Add turkey. Season to taste. Serve on rice and garnish with sprigs of parsley, lemon and tomato wedges. Serves 4.

Muffins

Total Calories	Starch Calories (Blocked by Starch-Blocker)	Non-starch Calories Remaining After Starch-Blocker Use	Ingredients
800	680	120	2 c. sifted flour
0	0	0	2 tsp. baking powder
0	0	0	½ tsp. salt
86	0	86	1⅓ T. honey
80	0	80	1 egg, beaten
90	0	90	1 c. skim milk
400	0	400	¼ c. melted shortening or oil
1,456	680	776	Totals per Recipe
121	56	65	Totals per Serving

Directions: Sift flour, baking powder, and salt together. Combine honey, egg, milk, and shortening. Add to the dry ingredients all at once. Mix only enough to moisten all the dry ingredients. Fill muffin pans (lined with paper liners or lightly greased) about two-thirds full. Bake at 375°-400° for 20 minutes or until top is lightly browned and springs back when touched. Makes 12.

Variations:

OATMEAL MUFFINS: Use 1 cup quick-cooking rolled oats instead of 1 cup of flour. This changes calorie count to:

1,430	580	850	Totals per Recipe
119	48	71	Totals per Serving

BLUEBERRY MUFFINS: Add 1 cup fresh blueberries. Reduce milk by ¼ cup and increase honey to 2⅔ T. This changes calorie count to:

1,665	800	865	Totals per Recipe
139	67	72	Totals per Serving

Liver and Rice Casserole

Total Calories	Starch Calories (Blocked by Starch-Blocker)	Non-starch Calories Remaining After Starch-Blocker Use	Ingredients
640	0	640	1 lb. calves liver, cubed
10	0	10	2 T. chopped celery
0	0	0	2 T. chopped green pepper
80	0	80	2 onions, sliced
140	0	140	2 T. whipped butter
340	0	340	2 c. tomato sauce
300	270	30	1½ c. cooked rice
0	0	0	½ tsp. salt, ¼ tsp. pepper
90	0	90	2 slices diced bacon, optional
1,600	270	1,330	Totals per Recipe
266	45	221	Totals per Serving

Directions: Saute celery, green pepper and onions in the butter. Add liver and cook over low heat until it changes color. Mix in tomato sauce, rice, salt and pepper. Place in buttered casserole, sprinkle with bacon, cover and bake for one hour in 350° oven. Serves 6.

Spaghetti . . . with Tomato Sauce or Sauce and Meatballs

Total Calories	Starch Calories (Blocked by Starch-Blocker)	Non-starch Calories Remaining After Starch-Blocker Use	Ingredients
690	240	450	3 cans (3 oz.) tomato paste
0	0	0	6 cans water
1,020	240	780	3 cans family-style tomato sauce (15-oz.)
276	80	196	1 46-oz. can tomato juice
50	0	50	1 onion, diced
0	0	0	salt and pepper
45	0	45	1 T. sugar
0	0	0	2 cloves garlic, minced
2,081	560	1,521	Totals per Recipe
104	28	76	Totals per Serving

Directions: Combine all ingredients, salt and peppering to taste. Bring to boil in large sauce pan, reduce heat and simmer for about six hours. Stir often to make sure it does not stick and burn on bottom. This makes enough sauce for 20 servings, and freezes very well. Simply pour the hot sauce over the cooked spaghetti, or serve separately—and always pass the grated Parmesan or Romano cheese for those not dieting. Serves 20.

Spaghetti . . . , cont.

If you want meat balls:

2,430	0	2,430	3 lbs. ground round steak
40	0	40	1 onion, diced
0	0	0	2 cloves garlic, diced
0	0	0	1 T. finely-ground anise seed
160	0	160	½ c. grated Romano cheese
240	0	240	3 eggs
2,870	0	2,870	Totals per Recipe
144	0	144	Totals per Serving

Directions: Mix all ingredients well. Shape in small meatballs. Brown in small amount of fat. Drop into hot tomato sauce and simmer together until meatballs are thoroughly cooked. Serves 20.

SPAGHETTI: One pound dry (1,680 calories) makes 6½ cups cooked at 190 calories per cup. Be sure and add this calorie count to your sauce when planning your menu.

Muffins

Total Calories	Starch Calories (Blocked by Starch-Blocker)	Non-starch Calories Remaining After Starch-Blocker Use	Ingredients
800	680	120	2 c. sifted flour
0	0	0	2 tsp. baking powder
0	0	0	½ tsp. salt
86	0	86	1⅓ T. honey
80	0	80	1 egg, beaten
90	0	90	1 c. skim milk
400	0	400	¼ c. melted shortening or oil
1,456	680	776	Totals per Recipe
121	56	65	Totals per Serving

Directions: Sift flour, baking powder, and salt together. Combine honey, egg, milk, and shortening. Add to the dry ingredients all at once. Mix only enough to moisten all the dry ingredients. Fill muffin pans (lined with paper liners or lightly greased) about two-thirds full. Bake at 375°-400° for 20 minutes or until top is lightly browned and springs back when touched. Makes 12.

Variations:

OATMEAL MUFFINS: Use 1 cup quick-cooking rolled oats instead of 1 cup of flour. This changes calorie count to:

1,430	580	850	Totals per Recipe
119	48	71	Totals per Serving

BLUEBERRY MUFFINS: Add 1 cup fresh blueberries. Reduce milk by ¼ cup and increase honey to 2⅔ T. This changes calorie count to:

1,665	800	865	Totals per Recipe
139	67	72	Totals per Serving

Liver and Rice Casserole

Total Calories	Starch Calories (Blocked by Starch-Blocker)	Non-starch Calories Remaining After Starch-Blocker Use	Ingredients
640	0	640	1 lb. calves liver, cubed
10	0	10	2 T. chopped celery
0	0	0	2 T. chopped green pepper
80	0	80	2 onions, sliced
140	0	140	2 T. whipped butter
340	0	340	2 c. tomato sauce
300	270	30	1½ c. cooked rice
0	0	0	½ tsp. salt, ¼ tsp. pepper
90	0	90	2 slices diced bacon, optional
1,600	270	1,330	Totals per Recipe
266	45	221	Totals per Serving

Directions: Saute celery, green pepper and onions in the butter. Add liver and cook over low heat until it changes color. Mix in tomato sauce, rice, salt and pepper. Place in buttered casserole, sprinkle with bacon, cover and bake for one hour in 350° oven. Serves 6.

Whole Wheat Noodles

Total Calories	Starch Calories (Blocked by Starch-Blocker)	Non-starch Calories Remaining After Starch-Blocker Use	Ingredients
800	680	120	2 c. whole wheat flour
160	0	160	2 eggs, large
10	0	10	2 T. skim milk
0	0	0	½ tsp. sea salt
970	680	290	Totals per Recipe
243	173	73	Totals per Serving

Directions: Combine all ingredients and knead for about 5 minutes. Sprinkle flour on bread board. Divide noodle mixture in half and roll each portion as thin as possible, turning rolled dough a couple of times during the rolling process. If you prefer, you can sprinkle some flour on the top of the rolled-out noodle dough and roll jelly-roll fashion, then cut and shake them out, or you can simply cut to desired width. These can be used at once, or you can spread them out and allow them to dry and store them in air-tight containers in freezer. Serves 4.

Bread Pudding

Total Calories	Starch Calories (Blocked by Starch-Blocker)	Non-starch Calories Remaining After Starch-Blocker Use	Ingredients
180	0	180	2 c. skim milk
160	0	160	2 eggs, beaten
660	600	60	2 c. slightly dry bread, cubed or torn
400	0	400	½ c. brown sugar
0	0	0	1 tsp. vanilla
0	0	0	pinch of salt
460	0	460	1 c. seedless raisins
0	0	0	1 tsp. cinnamon
1,860	600	1,260	Totals per Recipe
310	100	210	Totals per Serving

Directions: Place bread cubes in lightly buttered 8-inch square baking pan. Mix remainder of ingredients and pour them over the bread cubes. Place the baking dish in a larger pan in which there is about 1-inch of water. Bake at 375° for about 40 minutes or until a silver knife inserted in the center comes out clean. Serves 6.

Fruited Tapioca Parfait

Total Calories	Starch Calories (Blocked by Starch-Blocker)	Non-starch Calories Remaining After Starch-Blocker Use	Ingredients
133	113	20	⅓ c. minute tapioca
520	0	520	½ c. honey
100	0	100	2 c. fruit (fresh apples thinly sliced, raspberries or peaches)
0	0	0	2 c. water
0	0	0	2 T. lemon juice
0	0	0	½ tsp. nutmeg or cinnamon (optional)
0	0	0	pinch of salt
753	113	640	Totals per Recipe
188	28	160	Totals per Serving

Directions: Mix all ingredients and let stand for about 5 minutes. Bring to a boil, stirring often. Simmer until fruit is tender (about 10 minutes for apples and 8 for peaches and raspberries). Pour into parfait glasses. Serve warm or chilled. Serves 4.

Campfire Cornbread

Total Calories	Starch Calories (Blocked by Starch-Blocker)	Non-starch Calories Remaining After Starch-Blocker Use	Ingredients
570	480	90	1½ c. white corn meal, coarse stone ground
100	0	100	2 T. blackstrap molasses
0	0	0	1 tsp. salt
0	0	0	1 tsp. baking soda
160	0	160	2 eggs, well beaten
180	0	180	2 c. buttermilk
150	0	150	1½ T. melted margarine
1,160	480	680	Totals per Recipe
145	60	85	Totals per Serving
97	40	57	Totals per Small Serving

Directions: Heat oven to 400 degrees and place a 12-inch iron skillet or "spider" (an old iron skillet with legs which pioneers used so they could place the skillet over a bed of hot coals) in it to heat. Mix corn meal, molasses, salt, and baking soda in a bowl. Combine beaten eggs and buttermilk. Stir into cornmeal mixture. Add melted butter and pour into the hot skillet which has been well greased. Bake about 30 minutes or until cornbread is well browned and toothpick inserted into center comes out clean. Serves 8-12.

Boston Brown Bread

Total Calories	Starch Calories (Blocked by Starch-Blocker)	Non-starch Calories Remaining After Starch-Blocker Use	Ingredients
1,050	900	150	2½ c. whole wheat flour
800	0	800	1 c. molasses
80	0	80	1 egg
115	0	115	2 T. shortening
380	320	60	½ c. cornmeal (yellow)
0	0	0	1 tsp. salt
0	0	0	1½ tsp. each baking soda and baking powder
158	0	158	1¾ c. buttermilk
230	0	230	raisins
2,813	1,220	1,593	Totals per Recipe
141	61	80	Totals per Serving

Directions: Combine egg, molasses and softened shortening and beat well. Mix dry ingredients and raisins and add these and the buttermilk to the first mixture. Mix well and divide batter between two well greased 1-quart molds. (If you don't have molds, use two 1 lb. coffee cans or four soup cans. Be sure to remove paper wrapping and grease the cans well.) Seal the molds or cans with aluminum foil and set on a rack in a deep kettle containing enough boiling water to reach about halfway up the sides of the molds. Cover and steam very gently for about 2 hours. Replace water, if necessary. Makes enough bread for about 20 small slices.

Sourdough Pancakes or Waffles

Total Calories	Starch Calories (Blocked by Starch-Blocker)	Non-starch Calories Remaining After Starch-Blocker Use	Ingredients
50	20	30	½ c. sourdough starter
0	0	0	1 c. warm water
160	0	160	2 eggs
0	0	0	1 tsp. soda
90	0	90	1 c. milk, skim
800	680	120	2 c. flour (approximate)
0	0	0	½ tsp. salt
86	0	86	1⅓ T. honey
1,186	0	486	Totals per Recipe
118	70	48	Totals per Serving

Directions: Mix starter, milk, water and flour in large bowl. Blend and let set at room temperature overnight. Just before you start making pancakes add eggs, sugar, salt and soda and mix well but do not beat. Cook as you would any other pancakes. Serves 10.

For Waffles: Same as above except add 2 T. cooking oil. Serves 5.

1,426	700	725	Totals per Recipe
285	140	145	Totals per Serving

Refrigerator Muffins

Total Calories	Starch Calories (Blocked by Starch-Blocker)	Non-starch Calories Remaining After Starch-Blocker Use	Ingredients
1,440	0	1,440	2 c. sugar
1,840	0	1,840	1 c. shortening
0	0	0	2 c. boiling water
800	720	80	4 c. Kellogg's All-Bran
360	320	40	2 c. 100% Nabisco Bran
2,000	1,700	300	5 c. sifted flour
320	0	320	4 eggs, beaten
0	0	0	1 tsp. vanilla
0	0	0	5 tsp. baking soda
360	0	360	1 qt. buttermilk
0	0	0	1 tsp. salt
7,120	2,740	**42**	Totals per Recipe
109	42	**67**	Totals per Serving

Directions: Pour the hot water over the Nabisco Bran. Cream shortening with the sugar. Add Nabisco mixture, eggs, and buttermilk. Sift flour, soda and salt together and add all at once with Kellogg's All-Bran. Add vanilla. Fold only until all ingredients are moistened. Store in refrigerator in covered containers. Will keep six or seven weeks. Makes 1 gallon batter or about 65 muffins. Bake in greased muffin tins for 15 to 20 minutes in hot oven.

"My Own Favorite Starchy Recipes"

Total Calories	Starch Calories (Blocked by Starch-Blocker)	Non-starch Calories Remaining After Starch-Blocker Use	Ingredients (and amount)

Instructions:

(Photo copy this page to use for your favorite recipes.)

"My Own Favorite Starchy Recipes"

Total Calories	Starch Calories (Blocked by Starch-Blocker)	Non-starch Calories Remaining After Starch-Blocker Use	Ingredients (and amount)

Instructions:

(Photo copy this page to use for your favorite recipes.)

CHAPTER NINE

How To Begin Your Program

There is more to beginning the starch-blocker weight control program than to merely swallow a starch-blocker tablet. We recommend that all people who begin the program first fully familiarize themselves with the proper use of the product, that they tailor to themselves an individualized weight-loss and weight maintenance program, that they establish realistic goals for their weight loss, and that all significantly overweight people and anyone with a chronic health problem undergo a physical examination prior to beginning the program. We also recommend that people who feel that they eat compulsively contact an emotional counselor or a weight-loss peer-support group.

The surest way to fail on the starch-blocker weight loss program is to remain ignorant of what the starch-blocker can do—and what it can *not* do. Learning the parameters of the power of the starch-blocker assures a dieter of being able to properly use this powerful tool. Dieters who use the starch-blocker improperly will waste the best chance they have ever had to lose weight.

The best way to learn all about the starch-blocker is to read this book carefully, particularly the chapters on its use. These chapters will explain, for example, that dieters who expect the starch-blocker to block calories from foods other than starch, or who take it at the wrong time, are dieters who might as well not use this great new innovation.

We also urge dieters to learn all they can about the full scope of our program, because we think that it is extremely important for dieters beginning the program to appreciate the importance of dietary moderation, exercise, and the psychological aspects of overeating. If dieters enter the program thinking that this "wonder pill" will do all the work for them, they may never be successful weight-losers.

A dieter who exercises regularly will take off weight faster than an inactive dieter, and will be more likely to keep it off. Moderate daily exercise, as we've shown, can help you to lose up to one pound per week, in addition to the pounds that will be lost from caloric restriction and starch-blocking. But this weight, in turn, can be instantly regained through one binge of emotion-based gorging. We would very much like to see dieters become regular exercisers and emotionally-stable moderate-eaters.

In our technical society, which is oriented toward belief in the quick-fix and the easy-cure, people may try to endow the starch-blocker with powers it does not possess. People will probably want to think of the product as the "magic anti-fat pill," which it is not. The starch-blocker is, in actual fact, an amazingly helpful tool for those who use it in a carefully designed program, but it is *not* a magic cure-all. Dieters who are most familiar with the powers and the limitations of the product will be those who will be able to get the most good from it.

Plan to Lose!

A well-conceived plan, with realistic goals, can be greatly helpful to a person on a starch-blocker weight control program.

Dieters should begin this weight control program by choosing a "goal weight" for themselves. This goal weight should be realistic and achievable—nothing is more frustrating than struggling for an unattainable goal.

After setting their goal weights, dieters should calculate approximately how long they will have to stay in the weight loss phase of the weight control program, prior to shifting into the weight maintenance phase. Dieters may assume that they will lose several pounds per week, although the exact loss will vary greatly from dieter to dieter. Dieters will probably lose more weight in the earlier stages of their programs, when they have the most weight to lose.

Knowing approximately how long the weight loss phase of the program should last will probably make the experiencing of this phase somewhat easier—having an end in sight is almost always encouraging. The weight loss phase, of course, calls for a relatively low-calorie diet, so many dieters will be pleased when this phase ends. The weight maintenance phase, which the dieter begins once the goal weight is reached, allows an extremely rich, satisfying diet, so most people look forward to it.

After establishing a goal weight and a time-frame in which to reach it, dieters should devise a "meal plan," which can be either short-term or long-term, and can be either detailed or generalized.

People who enjoy planning and regimentation should plan an exact, strictly-ordered meal plan, while those who are most comfortable with flexibility may prefer a more loosely-structured plan. Both the careful plan and the loose plan can be equally helpful, depending upon one's preference.

A strict plan should list all the foods for all of the upcoming meals, including all snacks. The highly regimented plans may be helpful for dieters who are just beginning their weight control programs, because making it up can help dieters learn about caloric and starch contents. Dieters using the regimented plans should fill out the "Meal Plan Guide," included at the end of this chapter, in full detail, listing all of the foods they plan to eat (including all condiments, such as catsup and mayonnaise, which may be quite high in calories). Dieters can study the "Menu Plan" (found in the chapter "The Starch Blocker Diet"), as well as the "High-Starch Recipes" (also found in the chapter "The Starch Blocker Diet"), to help themselves plan interesting meals.

Minor digressions from the plan can be compensated for in later meals, of course, but dieters who use the detailed planning system should try not to stray very far from their original plans. If they do, there is no point in devising the strict meal plans. We advise against "cheating" on one's own plan, simply because it is human nature that occasional lapses tend to become frequent lapses, while strict adherence tends to remain strict adherence. Dieters should eat everything they have planned, but should not eat more than they have planned.

After several weeks of the strict plan, many dieters may choose to shift to the more loosely planned program. Some dieters, of course, will prefer to use the loosely planned program from the beginning. The loosely planned program can consist of only relatively vague meal plans, such as "chicken sandwich and salad," or "fish dinner with dessert." The food that is eaten, of course, must fall within the common sense guidelines of proper starch-blocker use. A "fish-dinner with dessert," for example, would have to consist of something like: broiled fish, a green salad, a baked potato, a dinner roll, a vegetable, and tapioca for dessert. It could not consist of deep-fried fish, a highly-sugared cole slaw, heavily buttered vegetables, and chocolate cake and ice cream. The high amounts of sugar and fat in the latter meal would be unaffected by the starch-blocker, and would pile on the pounds.

Most beginning dieters will find their weight control program much more effective if they use the detailed plan at first, then use the looser planning system after they have memorized the caloric and starch contents of various foods.

After knowledge of the starch and calorie contents of foods becomes second nature to dieters, they can abandon planning completely. This may take many months, however, and may never be a successful tactic for many dieters, including all of those who require a charting of food intake in order to keep from overeating.

An alternative to advance planning is keeping a diary of foods that have been eaten. This is essentially the same as planning, of course, except that it is done after the food is eaten, instead of before. By keeping a diary, a dieter is essentially free to plan meals on the spur of the moment, but still has a way of knowing when food intake is becoming excessive. Many dieters may shift from detailed planning to loose planning, and then to keeping a diary.

Some dieters who eventually abandon either keeping a diary or planning their diets may find it helpful to return to planning or keeping a diary if weight begins to creep back on.

We recommend that if a dieter has already shifted from specific planning to generalized planning before the weight maintenance phase is reached, that the dieter return to the specific planning routine when the maintenance phase is begun. The maintenance phase is considerably different from the weight loss phase, and requires a reorganization of one's eating habits. These eating habits are most easily influenced, we believe, by the practice of strict planning.

During all variation of planning, we urge dieters to include in their meal plans the foods they like most. If a dieter's favorite foods are high in sugar or fat, of course, these foods will have to be eaten in moderate amounts. But no food, as we have said before, is "forbidden." Even a food high in sugar and fat, such as ice cream, can be eaten occasionally. As dieters plan, they should search for high-starch recipes that they like, since starch calories, of course, can be blocked. Good starch recipes can be obtained from this book, or from many cookbooks.

When Medical Exams Are Needed

A full physical examination by a medical doctor should be necessary if the dieter who is about to begin the starch-blocker weight control program has a chronic health problem or is significantly overweight. By "significantly overweight," we refer to a dieter who is at least 20 percent over his or her proper weight; this would include, for example, a person who should weigh 100 pounds but actually weighs 120 pounds. It is always a good idea to have a checkup before starting any weight loss program.

People with chronic health problems would be those with any kind of heart condition, asthma, diabetes, arthritis, chronic infections or inflammations, emphysema, multiple sclerosis, etc. Any condition which is constantly annoying or which frequently requires medical attention indicates that a dieter should undergo a full physical examination before beginning the starch-blocker weight control program. We know of no particular reason why weight loss or dietary change would affect any chronic physical conditions, but because each person's metabolic and nutritional needs are different, a physical examination would be prudent for a person with a special problem. Nutrition often plays a part in many chronic disorders, and it would be unwise in some cases to tamper with one's nutritional balance.

We advise all dieters who are more than 20 percent

overweight to consult their physicians and receive a full physical examination prior to beginning our program, because high amounts of weight loss over a short time can sometimes be disruptive to general health. As a rule, weight loss in a significantly overweight person causes only positive benefits, but occasionally negative effects occur. One of the possible negative side-effects is stress to the kidneys brought on by the excretion of ketones (by-products from the burning of body-fat). A physical examination prior to beginning the program, with periodic check-ups, can help the significantly overweight dieter to avoid any possible negative effects from rapid weight-loss.

The examination should include a complete urinalysis, a complete blood test, an evaluation of medical history, and a physical work-up. It should also be remembered that many physicians are experts in nutrition and weight control, and the advice and care of these professionals can often cause the starch-blocker weight control program to reach its peak of effectiveness.

Special Help for Dieters

Some dieters should seek the help of physicians who specialize in nutrition, or the help of emotional counselors, or the help of weight-loss groups.

Not every dieter will be totally self-motivated. Many dieters do best when they receive the support of an expert or the support of the peers in their weight-loss group. Other dieters need the support of an emotional counselor to overcome the urge to overeat.

Only the individual truly knows if he or she will significantly benefit from the services of a supportive person or group. If you feel you might benefit from help, *don't be afraid to ask for it.*

Not every dieter will be able to successfully organize his or her entire weight control meal plan. People having difficulty should consult a doctor who works with nutrition. Some dieters will probably have questions that this book doesn't answer, and an expert on nutrition is the best source for answers to these questions.

Weight loss groups, such as Weight Watchers or T.O.P.S., can be very helpful to dieters who enjoy the camaraderie of group support. Sharing experiences, problems and aspirations is a considerable psychological stimulus to many people. In general, the starch-blocker weight control program's dietary recommendations are compatible with those of most of these groups, except that the starch-blocker program recommends, of course, more use of starchy foods. A modified Weight Watchers diet, perhaps with starchy foods added, could work very well as the dietary component of a starch-blocker weight control program. As we have said, we are not doctrinaire or dogmatic about what people choose for their diets, so long as these diets are devised with common sense and restraint. Any balanced, relatively low-fat, low-sugar diet will provide a sufficient base for the starch-blocker weight control program.

Starting Your Program

Once you have made a commitment to lose weight, have fully familiarized yourself with the starch-blocker, have planned your program, and have gotten a physical examination if you have a special health problem, you are ready to begin your program.

If you have prepared properly, you will stand a superb chance of putting the powerful tool of the starch-blocker to its best possible use. And if the starch-blocker is put to its best use, you will probably achieve your goal—a new, slim figure, one that will still be here next month, and next year, and the year after. And for the rest of your life.

THE MEAL PLAN GUIDE

Food	Amount	Calories	Blocked Starch Calories	Remaining Calories In Food After Starch-blocker Use
EXAMPLE:				
Breakfast:				
Bread	2 pieces	220	200	20
Eggs	2	160	0	160
Potatoes	1 medium	120	100	20
Butter	1 Tablespoon	50	0	50
		550 Total Calories	300 Total Blocked Starch Calories	250 Total Remaining Calories
Snack:				
Lunch:				
Snack:				
Dinner:				
Snack:				

THE MEAL PLAN GUIDE

Food	Amount	Calories	Blocked Starch Calories	Remaining Calories In Food After Starch-blocker Use
Breakfast:				
Snack:				
Lunch:				
Snack:				
Dinner:				
Snack:				

(You may photocopy this page.)

THE MEAL PLAN GUIDE

Food	Amount	Calories	Blocked Starch Calories	Remaining Calories In Food After Starch-blocker Use
Breakfast:				
Snack:				
Lunch:				
Snack:				
Dinner:				
Snack:				

(You may photocopy this page.)

PART FOUR

Why You Didn't Lose Before— And Why You Should Now

CHAPTER TEN

What's Wrong with Other Diets

In the early 1950s, a self-styled diet promoter named a diet after one of America's most prestigious medical clinics—without that clinic's consent. This diet inaugurated the past thirty years of dietary inanity. The promoter of the diet claimed that dieters should shovel down all the fatty meat they wanted and still lose weight. This relatively ridiculous "famous clinic diet" was one of the first nationally popular, media-promoted weight-loss diets. The diet created a model that a great many diets have since mimicked. The model consists of diets that are: (1) nutritionally unsound; (2) ineffective at achieving permanent weight loss; (3) promoted cleverly in the mass media; and (4) enormously popular for a short time. In short, the diet was the first of what are now commonly called "fad diets."

From this 1950s "famous clinic diet" to today's "famous suburb diets," fad diets have regularly emerged that promise dieters a weight loss that will be *fast! easy!!* and *permanent!!!* Most of these fad diets, which are generally championed by diet gurus with more experience in public relations than nutrition, are absolutely ridiculous. Some of them contain a kernel of common sense.

A few dietary regimes have been proposed, however, that are based on long-term reduced-calorie eating plans. These regimes actually offer sound, sensible advice.

The diets offering this good advice are those that merely recommend cutting excessive carbohydrates and fats from the diet. These low-calorie diets are generally the types recommended by the reputable weight loss groups, such as Weight Watchers or T.O.P.S. The only problem with these low-calorie diets, though, is that they are generally hard for a dieter to stick to, especially if the dieter does not regularly have the encouragement of his or her peer support group. Our hope, of course, is that the starch-blocker will make these nutritionally sound, low-calorie diets a great deal easier, by allowing the eating of many more starchy foods that will never be processed as calories.

Nothing, however, could make easy some of the diets that have been promoted over the past thirty years. Ever since the birth of the first "famous clinic diet," an endless parade of fad diets has marched past our overweight population, with each diet in the parade seductively cooing: "Try me! I'm easy!" But none of them are.

Mono Diet Mania

Diets like the first "famous clinic diet," which restrict the dieter to eating only *one* food, are not only nutritionally unsound and ineffective as weight loss programs, but are also *far from easy*. The "famous clinic diet," and many like it, are basically just "mono" diets—diets based on the eating of a single food. However hard the promoters of these diets may try to sell the "easiness" of these eating plans, the fact remains that there is nothing easy about trying to live on only one food.

Even if that food is a relatively good food, available in many varieties—such as the meat that composes most of the "famous clinic diet"—restriction of a diet to primarily or only one food will invariably become boring, and will also quite possibly result in nutritional imbalances. Many different foods have been featured in the various varieties of mono diets that have been promoted. Gracing the history of nutritional science are the Grapefruit Diet, the Ice Cream Diet, the Banana Diet, the Candy Diet and the Rice Diet. Some of these mono-diet foods were said to exert special powers—grapefruits, for example, were alleged to have a special "fat-burning" enzyme, and ice cream was said to coat the intestines, blocking calorie absorption. The scientific evidence supporting these assertions was always slim, however. All any of these mono diets ever really did, in reality, was to simply make the dieter tired of eating the *one food* that was allowed—causing a natural cessation of eating. By this line of reasoning, dieters might be well advised to merely smear all of their food with bear-grease—that action would also reduce one's appetite!

But after dieters got tired of eating bear-greased food, of course, they would probably return to the same fattening diet that they had been eating before. And that, needless to say, is exactly what happens to dieters on a mono diet. After bananas or ice cream start to "come out their ears," dieters tend to fall back into the same eating patterns that had caused their overweight condition in the first place. At the end of their mono diet, they may be a few pounds heavier or they may be a few pounds lighter, depending upon how much of their mono-food they ate. But they will also quite possibly be deficient in a number of nutrients, and these nutritional deficiencies may well trigger hunger. A person coming off an all-grapefruit diet, for example, might have a protein shortage that would cause a craving for meat, and possible over-eating of meat. The mono diets are notorious for precipitating the "yo-yo" effect of fat/thin, fat/thin. Luckily, the obvious foolishness of trying to live off just grapefruits or ice cream has enabled the majority of dieters over the past thirty years to not take most mono diets very seriously. Unfortunately, though, some mono-oriented diets, patterned after the original "famous clinic diet," have been promoted very skillfully by a few doctors, and have gained credibility in the minds of many people. These diets are the low-carbohydrate, high-protein diets that have spawned the spurious notion that "calories don't count."

Calories Do Count

In the 1970s, a doctor-author with immense media-savvy proposed the idea that calories don't count, as long as these calories come from protein rather than from carbohydrates (starch and sugar). This "low carbohydrate" diet has dominated much of the last decade.

The usual concept in weight loss, of course, is that the only way to lose pounds of stored food energy, otherwise known as fat, is to burn up more food than you take in. Because "calorie" is a measure of food energy, it is assumed that the only way to lose weight is to decrease caloric intake, or to increase caloric use.

Calories can be eaten as proteins, fats, or carbohydrates. Carbohydrates are the easiest foods to digest, and provide much of our food energy. Proteins can substitute for carbohydrates if necessary, and this action is used in low-carbohydrate diets.

The low-carbohydrate diet, which originated as the "famous clinic diet," was hotly promoted, and later "canonized," in two blockbuster bestsellers by the doctor-author. The low-carbohydrate diet is based on the dubious notion that one can eat almost all the high-protein, low-carbohydrate foods that one wants and still lose weight.

One is supposed to be able to lose weight, the diet doctor says, because a fat-mobilizing substance will miraculously appear if one eats plenty of fat. The diet doctor recommends that dieters eat all the bacon and eggs they can stuff down, while curtailing their intake of fruits, vegetables, and grains. The famous diet doctor says a person can eat 4,000 to 5,000 calories of non-carbohydrate foods each day and still lose weight, because one's body will become a fat-burning machine. No laboratory evidence has confirmed this claim, and the AMA Council on Nutrition has voiced "deep concern" about this diet. But this best-selling diet doctor is currently one of the best-known diet "authorities" in the nation, lending impressive testimony to the concept that people will believe anything, so long as it's good news.

Another diet guru who has captivated the media and public recently is the creator of the famed "liquid protein" diet. But this doctor's diet is not even really a mono diet; it is merely a fast accompanied by protein supplementation, which keeps the body from burning muscle tissue. The diet was investigated by the FDA as the possible culprit in thirty-six deaths due to a mineral imbalance that disturbed heartbeat rhythm. It's hard to deny that this diet works: if you don't eat, you're bound to lose weight. But like any other crash diet, this one beckons the "yo-yo effect."

This diet doctor claims in his best-selling book that 80 percent of all people who use this diet never regain the weight lost on the diet. He also admits, though, that "no data exists yet for claims of success that are medically meaningful."

It is our belief that no data proving bold claims on this diet's powers will *ever* emerge, because the possible success of this diet goes against the grain of everything we know about weight loss. It is simply impossible for us to believe that a dieter will maintain weight loss after a crash diet. And a total fast, even one in which protein is poured down the throat, is certainly the ultimate crash diet.

The Latest Fads

Two recent fad diets which captured millions of people's hearts and minds—if not their fat—were the highly celebrated "fruit sugar diet" and the mega-hyped, famous-suburb "pineapple diet."

The fruit sugar diet purports to offer dieters a way to "turn off" their "hunger alarm switch." This rather mysterious "hunger alarm switch," which apparently is nothing more than a gimmicky name for hunger, is supposed to be switched off with pure fruit sugar, or fructose. Most doctors and nutritionists, of course, think that eating fruit sugar is an ineffective way to lose weight; in fact, they associate eating any kind of sugar with *gaining* weight. The fruit sugar diet's primary promoter, though, suggests taking a few fructose tablets with one's meal, to depress the appetite. This strategy seems substantially similar to that proposed by the sellers of "diet candies," the sugary morsels that are supposed to kill appetites.

The fruit sugar diet, then, is nothing more than a low-calorie diet that is supplemented with fructose. This starkly simplistic weight loss plan became extremely popular for a couple of years, as it was relentlessly flogged on talk show after talk show.

Even more aggressively marketed, though, was the famous-suburb, movie-star-endorsed "pineapple diet," which was conceived of by a person who has virtually no formal training in nutrition or any other biological science. This person culled the basic idca for this frighteningly successful diet from some antique health-food books that she happened to read.

The major thesis of the diet is that different foods require different pancreatic enzymes for digestion, and that if certain foods are eaten simultaneously, digestion will be somewhat more difficult, because the pancreas will be called upon to produce many enzymes at once. This is a true enough assertion. The diet impressario's assertions stray into the realm of whimsy, however, when it is claimed that poorly digested foods get "stuck in the stomach" and "turn into fat." The claim that "undigested" food causes weight gain, of course, contradicts the very meaning of the word "digest," which implies the process of adding food energy, or calories, to the body. This indulgence in yarn-spinning has earned this diet's creator the scorn of even non-medical publications such as *People* magazine, which has quoted an authority to the effect that the "pineapple diet" is "nonsensical nutritional gobbledygook."

In order to keep this "stuck food" from "turning into fat," the diet guru recommends that people eat nothing but fruit, and especially pineapple, for three weeks, then go on a diet very high in fruit. The fruit meals are interspersed with meals that do not appear to be terribly weighted toward nutritional balance—consider, for example, the nutritional qualities of a dinner of "pasta and vodka," or a dinner solely composed of "popcorn."

It may be true that going on a fruit fast will help a person to lose weight, but the diet's creator tries to foist off this limited dietary regime as a lifelong eating plan. She even has the gall to call the diet "fun." How can it be "fun," though, to eat nothing all day long except "grapes" for breakfast, nothing for lunch, and "two glasses of wine" for dinner? To us, this sounds like slow starvation. This diet may be a fairly effective way to crash one's weight down for a *Vogue* magazine modeling assignment, but it certainly doesn't appear to be an "easy" diet. The diet, in fact, is difficult to follow, and like any other very low protein diet, it threatens a shortage of the mineral potassium, which can cause heartbeat rhythms to become so disrupted that death can occur. A U.C.L.A. endoctrinologist has called the "pineapple diet" a "disaster waiting to happen." The diet's promoter has shown little public concern about either the essential ineffectiveness of her diet as a long-term eating plan, or about the possibly fatal biochemical imbalances the diet may cause. Instead, she continues to blithely hype the diet as the "cure for fat." Following in the footsteps of other diet hucksters, she feels no apparent qualms about employing the well-worn claims of *"fast!"*, *"easy!!"*, and *"permanent!!!"*, which still seem to strike a responsive chord in overweight people.

The fact is, though, that almost *nothing* that is fast and easy *ever* seems to be permanent. We do not claim that the starch-blocker weight loss program is necessarily fast and easy. It *can* work quickly as a weight loss program, *if* the dieter *makes* it work quickly. It also may be easier than other weight control programs, because of the use of the starch-blocker. But it is *not* as easy as eating anything one wants. And the starch-blocker program may indeed cause a permanent weight loss, but this loss will only be permanent if the dieter *makes* it permanent.

The Reasonable Diets

Not all diets that have been proposed over the past thirty years, thank goodness, have been irresponsible and over-sold. Some have been sensible. Diets that call for a moderate reduction of caloric intake over a long period of time are sensible, effective weight loss devices. Calories do count; they are responsible for all weight that is gained. Some people, because of their metabolism or degrees of physical activity, are able to eat more than others without gaining weight. All people who do gain weight, though, gain it because they are eating more calories than is appropriate for their activity levels and metabolisms.

The best ways to block calories are to limit the eating of fat and sugar, and to block starch calories with the starch-blocker. The first sensible diets were not able to use the starch-blocker, of course, so they relied upon avoiding fat and sugar. The first of the responsible diets was the Prudent Diet, created in 1957 by Dr. Norman Joliffe of the New York City Health Department. Dr. Joliffe's diet has been imitated by many other low-calorie diets over twenty-five years, including the Weight Watcher's Diet, the Air Force Diet, and the T.O.P.S. Diet.

The Prudent Diet limits calories to about 2,400 per day, which is substantially lower than the approximately 3,200 daily calories eaten by the average American. Even 2,400 calories, though, may be more than many people need, so this diet is not perfect.

Dr. Joliffe recommended that people lower their intake of fat. Most people eat about 42 percent of their calories as fat; Dr. Joliffe recommended they lower fat intake to account for 35 percent of all calories.

The Prudent Diet is essentially just a well-balanced diet, high in fruits, vegetables, and lean meat. The diet is not a crash diet or a fad diet. It is, rather, a reasonable eating program that a well-disciplined person could maintain indefinitely. It may call for too many calories for some people, but will be appropriate for others.

The reputable weight loss groups, such as Weight Watchers, use a basic Prudent Diet, but translate the calories into "portions" and "units" to make it easier for the dieter to plan meals. The diets of these weight loss groups are, as a rule, good eating plans that could be maintained throughout a life-time by a dedicated dieter.

As reasonable as these low-calorie diets are, however, a great many people cannot seem to stay with them. The low calorie diets often do not offer the taste appeal, bulk and variety that most people love. Therefore, it has been quite common for dieters who are somewhat undisciplined to stray from even the most reasonable of the balanced, low-calorie eating plans.

Now, however, that dieters can employ the starch-blocker to enrich and enliven these reasonable diets, a whole new era in dieting has begun.

The reasonable diets, combined with the use of the starch-blocker, will provide dieters with a path to fitness and slimness that never before existed.

CHAPTER ELEVEN

Why It's Important To Lose Weight

Being overweight is as harmful to you as you have always suspected it is. Overweight people die younger, have less energy, and according to health experts and the U.S. government, are excessively prone to heart disease, cancer, diabetes and other diseases.

Being overweight has a great many drawbacks and virtually no advantages. It is a formidable threat to your ability to enjoy life—and even to your ability to continue to live.

Fat vs. Health

Between one-fourth to one-half of all Americans are digging their graves with their forks. They are carrying an extra burden of unhealthful, unattractive fat with them everywhere they go. The only compensation they receive is that the more weight they have to carry, the shorter time they are apt to have to carry it.

A general rule of thumb, accepted by many bariatric physicians (doctors who specialize in weight reduction), is that people shorten their lives by approximately the same percentage that they are over their ideal weights—for example, people who are 10 percent overweight will be likely to have their lives shortened by about 10 percent. In other words, a person with a normal life expectancy of 70—who weighs 110 pounds when he or she should weigh 100—will be likely to die seven years earlier than expected, or age 63.

By this same reasoning, people who are 20 percent overweight will probably cut 20 percent off their lifespans, and people who are 50 percent overweight may cut their lives in half! Dr. Rene Dubos, author of many books on health, summarizes the situation: "History repeats itself. Like the prosperous Romans of 2,000 years ago, many prosperous citizens of the Western world today dig their own graves through overeating."

Fat and Your Heart

Heart disease is one of the diseases most closely related to being overweight. Cardiovascular conditions that are linked to overweight include high blood pressure, hardening of the arteries, and the clogging of the arteries with fatty deposits. These conditions cause heart attacks and strokes.

Being overweight causes many stresses to the entire cardiovascular system. When people become overweight, extra fat deposits all over the body require extra blood circulation, taxing the heart. The heart also becomes covered with a heavy coating of fatty tissue, which makes its pumping action more difficult to perform. Also, the heart is likely to be pushed out of its normal position by fat deposits in the abdominal and thoracic cavities; the heart tends to be pushed upward toward the neck by these collections of fat, where its ability to perform normally is further diminished.

It is not completely understood why the arteries and vessels become hardened and inelastic in overweight people. The hardened condition is believed to stem, though, from a general deterioration of the tissues that make up blood vessels. The vessels also become narrowed on the inside as fat clings to their walls. These narrow vessels, with little elasticity, cause an increase in the pressure of the circulatory system, just as the water pressure in a garden hose is increased if the hose is squeezed. This combination of factors—narrowed veins, clogged veins, high pressure, a heart covered with fat, a heart out of its normal position, and a body with many extra pounds requiring circulation—often proves to be a fatal combination for overweight people. Each of these conditions tends to aggravate the other conditions in this circulatory "chain" of many "weak links."

Often the first "weak link" in the "chain" to break is the heart muscle itself. If the artery that supplies the heart with blood becomes blocked, the heart stops, often causing death by heart attack. Another very common occurrence is a blockage of blood to the brain, which can also be caused by hardened, fat-clogged vessels; when this happens, a person can die or be disabled by a "stroke." There are other fatal cardiovascular diseases, but heart attack and stroke are by far the most common.

People who are not overweight also die of cardiovascular diseases, of course, but these diseases are about 150 percent higher in overweight people, and increase in likelihood with every extra pound of fat that is added. About one-half of all people die of cardiovascular diseases.

Fat and Diabetes

Diabetes is even more closely linked to a condition of overweight than are cardiovascular diseases. Diabetes is about 400 percent more common in overweight people than slim people. Diabetes is characterized by excessive sugar in the blood, a condition caused by insufficient production of insulin, which helps transfer sugar out of the blood and into the cells. Diabetes can generally be controlled with diet, and/or insulin injections, or other medications, but can cause low resistance to infections, blindness, cardiovascular diseases and metabolic disorders. Control of diabetes is much more difficult in significantly overweight people, and is considered incurable in all people.

It is suspected that the high-sugar and high-starch foods often eaten by overweight people contribute to the onset of diabetes. Sugary foods, and food high in starch—which is quickly converted into blood sugar—stress the digestive abilities of the pancreas, which produces insulin.

Another vital organ that is taxed by the type of diet associated with a condition of overweight, and with excessive body fat itself, is the liver. Cirrhosis of the liver is about 250 percent more common in overweight people than in thin people. When a person is overweight, the liver, which helps to digest food and helps to clean the blood, can swell to 150 percent its normal size. Fat deposits push the swollen liver into the lung cage, further disturbing its function. When people eat excessively, their livers are forced to produce digestive secretions in abnormal quantities, which can exhaust this important organ. The liver itself can become fatty, which further inhibits its ability to function properly. A poorly functioning liver not only makes digestion more difficult, but can cause problems throughout the entire system, as the liver's failure to clean the blood produces general toxic overload. A non-functioning liver, of course, causes death.

Fat and Cancer

Cancer is also more common in overweight people. The federal government's National Cancer Institute has issued a warning that a condition of overweight will make a person more vulnerable to all forms of cancer in general, and especially vulnerable to certain forms of cancer, such as uterine cancer in women.

As long ago as 1959, it was shown that overweight people die of cancer more frequently than do thin people, and that the more overweight a person is, the more likely he or she will be to die from cancer. In 1959, Dr. Albert Tannenbaum, in *The Physiology of Cancer,* demonstrated, through studies of large population groups, that men who were overweight by 25 percent or more had a cancer death rate that was 30 percent higher than that of men whose weights were normal.

It was later shown that some cancers, such as uterine cancer, were 300 percent to 900 percent more common in overweight women. Other cancers that are believed to be associated with a condition of overweight are cancers of the breast, colon, prostate, ovary and pancreas. These cancers are so closely related to overeating that they are referred to by Dr. John Berg of the Cancer Epidemiology Research Center of the University of Iowa as cancers of "affluent nutrition."

It is theorized that a condition of overweight influences cancer causation by disrupting hormonal balance. It is also believed that the eating patterns associated with being overweight, including high consumption of sugar and fat, have direct adverse effects upon the organs of digestion and elimination, such as the pancreas and colon. Dr. Donald Germann, a researcher of diet-related cancers, has written in *The Anti-Cancer Diet* that "the correlation between breast cancer, colon cancer and fat intake . . . is positively breathtaking."

Fat, Arthritis and Fatigue

Other health problems associated with being overweight are arthritis, back pain, and chronic fatigue.

The link between being overweight and having arthritis is a tentative one, but the disease is more common in overweight people, according to arthritis specialist Collin H. Dong, M.D., of San Francisco. Dr. Dong believes that some of the foods associated with being overweight, and particularly sugar, irritate the joints of persons with arthritis. He believes certain high-fat and high-sugar foods cause metabolic disruption and allergic reaction. Dr. Dong treats arthritis with a regime that revolves around dietary change. It is obvious, of course, that extra weight puts extra stress on joints that support the body, such as the knees and ankles.

A somewhat similar disease, gout, can be controlled by lowering sugar, fat and alcohol intake. Gout, which over one million people in North America suffer from, has long been identified as a disease related to eating excess quantities of rich foods.

The strain on the back muscles and skeletal system caused by the pull of excess pounds can cause chronic back pain. A condition of overweight causes structural imbalance, pulling the body out of its normal center of gravity. The structural stress caused by being overweight can also aggravate muscles, joints and tendons throughout the body.

General fatigue is a final health problem associated with being overweight. A person who must always carry around twenty or thirty extra pounds—the equivalent of a heavy backpack—is under a constant physical strain. Complicating the situation is the fact that this extra burden of weight must be carried by a body that has decreased circulatory and respiratory abilities. Lung capacity, for example, may be reduced by as much as one-third in the body of an overweight person. Metabolic problems, such as hypoglycemia or a pre-diabetic condition, may further sap the overweight person's energy.

Being overweight, then, is not just a threat to long-term health, but is a constant, day-in, day-out irritation to the entire body.

A final consideration is the emotional stress that can be caused by all of these various negative health factors. Physical ailments are among the most mentally disturbing of all of life's problems. This emotional turmoil can, in turn, create a desire to over-eat. Clearly, a vicious circle of "overeating/ill health/emotional upset/and further over-eating" can be created.

It is important that you recognize the danger of this vicious circle—and work hard to stay *healthy* and *happy.*

Furthermore, it is important that you recognize the general threat to health that being overweight poses. Although you may be primarily concerned about how being overweight makes you *look,* you should not ignore how being overweight can make you *feel.*

PART FIVE

Answers and Interviews

CHAPTER TWELVE

Answers To Your Questions

It seems as if most dieters we have talked to have asked essentially the same questions. Therefore, we have kept a list of the most-asked questions and have compiled them in the following dialogue format.

Q. I don't eat very much, but I'm still overweight. Why?

A. Regardless of the exact quantity of food you have been eating, there is no doubt that you have been eating more food than your body can metabolize as energy. The potential energy that is in food, which is quantified as "calories," is metabolized immediately as energy, or is stored for later energy, either in the liver, the muscles—or as fat. You have, therefore, eaten more "food energy" than you have used, even though the amount you have eaten seems relatively small to you. The only way to reverse your situation of overweight is to metabolize less *food energy* than your body needs for its *physical energy*. If you do this, your body will burn its "stored energy," including, of course, your fat. You can metabolize less either by eating fewer calories, or by blocking calories from starch with the starch-blocker.

Q. But other people seem to eat more than I do without "storing" their foods as fat. How can I be like them?

A. You can't—you can only be "like you." Many other people may have a more efficient, "faster" metabolism than you, one which has a natural tendency to use food energy rather than to store it. These people will be able to eat more food than you without gaining weight. Many other people, though, may have a "slower" metabolism than you. More than likely, you are in the "average" range in metabolic efficiency. Most people *do* metabolize their food approximately equally. Only about three percent of all people really have serious metabolic problems that make them gain weight extremely easily.

You should consider the possibility that you actually *do* eat more calories than people who seem to eat less than you. Perhaps you eat less quantity than them, but eat higher calorie foods, such as sweets or fatty meat. Fat contains over twice as many calories per ounce as protein or carbohydrates. Perhaps you eat small amounts at meals, but snack frequently. Or perhaps you are much less physically active than people who seem to eat more than you, but who weigh less. No matter why you are overweight, though, there is really only one solution to the problem—you must begin to use more food energy than you absorb as calories. We recommend that you do this by using the starch-blocker weight control program, which is a combination of increased exercise, a careful diet, and use of the starch-blocker.

Q. But I've tried *so many* different diets that I've become skeptical of all of them. Do you think any of them really work?

A. Many of them work—for a short time. Any diet that restricts caloric intake will probably cause a weight loss. The problem with diets is not that they don't work, but that few people can stay with them. Most people have been able to lose weight on various diets, but haven't been able to *maintain* the weight loss because the diet is too boring or unfulfilling. Only about four percent of all people now on a weight control diet are on a diet for the first time—the other 96 percent of all dieters have tried other diets that have not resulted in long-term success.

Q. How does the starch-blocker weight control program avoid this problem?

A. It avoids it by using a nutritional dietary aid that hasn't been employed in any other weight control program. That nutritional substance, of course, is the starch-blocker. The starch-blocker keeps starch from being absorbed as calories, and therefore enables the dieter to eat a more varied, satisfying diet. Because dieters can eat an interesting, fulfilling diet, they are much less likely to stray from the diet. Being able to eat a fulfilling diet, without gaining weight, is, after all, what most dieters have been wishing for all of their lives.

Q. Do special foods have to be eaten on your program?

A. No. The average person normally eats about 25 percent of his or her diet as starch. If the starch-blocker were used regularly, and no adjustments were made in this average diet, the person would still remove about 25 percent of all calories from the diet. If, however, a person consciously switched to a diet higher in starch content, then an even greater percentage of all calories eaten would be blocked. If a person began eating lots of potatoes and bread and rice and pasta, which are high in starch, he or she might be able to block 35 to 40 percent of all calories from the diet. A special, high-starch diet can be used, then, but it is not necessary. The best diet to eat with the starch-blocker is a balanced, wholesome, moderate diet, low in fat and sugar.

Q. Does the starch-blocker have any effect on foods other than starch?

A. None whatsoever. Besides being composed of starch, food is composed of protein, sugar and fat, none of which are affected by the starch-blocker. Vitamins and minerals are also unaffected by the starch-blocker.

Q. Does that mean that if you ate a piece of bread, you would get all the proteins, fats, sugars and vitamins and minerals from the bread, but just not the starch?

A. Exactly.

Q. But doesn't your body need the starch?

A. No, starch isn't an essential nutrient. It merely provides energy, which can also be derived from sugars, fats and proteins. We advise people on the starch-blocker weight control program to rely primarily upon proteins for their food energy. Proteins are preferable to sugars and fats because they provide the body with many "building materials." Proteins are also preferable because sugars are disruptive to the metabolism, and fats contain more calories per ounce than other food components, and can be difficult to digest.

Q. What kinds of foods contain starch?

A. Starch is found in almost all foods that come from the plant kingdom—grains, fruits and vegetables. Foods that are *very* high in starch are potatoes, breads, pasta, spaghetti, beans, corn, rice, cereals, and some fruits. If these foods are eaten with the starch-blocker, most of the calories in them will never be absorbed in the body.

Q. What exactly is the starch-blocker?

A. The starch-blocker is a natural, organic protein substance extracted from kidney beans. It is pure, non-toxic, easy to use, and is available in tablet form.

Q. What does it do?

A. The effect of the starch-blocker is simple and limited. It nutritionally inhibits the action of alpha amylase, the digestive enzyme that changes starch into glucose (blood sugar), which is then used by the body as calories. Changing starch into calories is the only function of this enzyme. When the enzyme is stopped from "doing its job," the starch you eat is not converted into calories, and ultimately into fat.

Q. How does the starch-blocker work?

A. Let's say you eat a potato, a good, nutritious food, but one high in starch calories. Along with the potato, you take a starch-blocker tablet. In the body, all the nutrients of the potato—the vitamins, minerals and other nutrients—are digested and absorbed normally. But the starch—essentially "empty" calories—is not digested and absorbed. About 80 to 90 percent of the caloric content of the potato comes from starch, so you get all of the important nutrition, but very few of the calories.

Q. But why doesn't the starch-blocker affect all the other foods that I eat?

A. Proteins, fats, and sugars are digested by *other* enzymes. Vitamins, minerals and other nutrients reach the body through other pathways.

Q. How much starch will one starch-blocker tablet block?

A. You can expect one tablet to block up to 100 grams (or 3½ ounces) of pure starch, which is the equivalent of 400 calories. This is more starch than is eaten at an average meal. So one tablet at an average meal should be adequate to block the meal's starch calories.

Q. Is the starch-blocker safe?

A. Yes. People with known food allergies to beans, however, should use the starch-blocker with discretion, since it is derived from kidney beans.

It is normal to experience an increased feeling of bulk or fullness, due to the passage of undigested starch. Drinking adequate fluids facilitates this passage. This increased bulk is beneficial to dieters, since dieters tend to lack dietary bulk due to decreased food consumption.

A few people are aware of minor bloating or gas, which usually disappears after a few days of starch-blocker use.

Because the starch-blocker is a natural substance, with such a limited activity, it causes no unusual physical effects. This has been proven in tests, studies and experiments over several years. The starch-blocker remains in the digestive tract. Unlike weight-loss aids such as appetite suppressants, diuretics and stimulants, the starch-blocker does not cause feelings of fatigue or irritated nerves. The starch-blocker is a special food for dietary use, and is safe and not habit-forming.

Q. When was the starch-blocker discovered?

A. The starch-blocker was first discovered over ten years ago and has been painstakingly developed and tested ever since.

Q. What do the tests on the starch-blocker show?

A. They show that it is as safe as it is effective. Extensive tests on laboratory animals proved the product has remarkable abilities to nutritionally inhibit starch digestion, and is nontoxic. After the product was perfected, studies with people conducted by weight clinics showed that people using the starch-blocker was able to effectively inhibit the digestion of starch that was eaten. In those tests, people were able to eat substantially more than another group of dieters who weren't using the starch-blocker.

Q. Do you need a doctor to supervise your use of the starch-blocker?

A. No, but you may wish to have a doctor who is knowledgeable about nutrition help you design a diet that will provide all the nutrients you need for good health. If you eat a gross excess of starchy foods while taking the starch-blocker, you may not get a well-balanced diet.

Q. Can anyone take the starch-blocker?

A. Almost anyone can. However, for the sake of caution, we recommend the starch-blocker not be used by pregnant women, or by people with special metabolic problems, such as diabetes. Pregnancy is generally not a very good time for a weight-control diet, and no tests have yet been conducted with diabetics using the starch-blocker.

Q. Because the starch-blocker doesn't affect sugars or fats, will I have to be moderate in eating sweets and high-fat foods?

A. Yes. Don't get carried away with hot-fudge sundaes and fried foods, because these foods will still make you fat. These foods, obviously, are not high in starch, and are loaded with calories from fat and sugar.

Q. What foods are highest in starch?

A. A few of them are: beans, peas, corn, potatoes, squash, bananas, barley, biscuits, bread, cornflakes, macaroni, noodles, rice, spaghetti and tapioca. There are many more, and most are good, nutritious foods.

Q. How should I take the starch-blocker?

A. One tablet should be taken immediately prior to any meal or snack containing up to 400 calories from starch, if you wish to block those starch calories. The tablet should be taken just before food is eaten; it does not inhibit starch digestion if taken *between meals or snacks*.

Q. How will I know the starch-blocker is working?

A. After a few days, look at the scale! One note—the first few days after using the starch-blocker, you may actually gain a little weight. This is because the undigested starch tends to absorb water while in the digestive tract. This will very quickly go away.

Q. How long should I continue to use the starch-blocker?

A. For as long as you wish to block starch calories.

After you achieve a desired weight, you may not need to continue using it. You may, however, want to use it occasionally, particularly with very starchy meals, to help maintain your desired weight.

CHAPTER THIRTEEN

Interviews with Starch-Blocker Users

The following are sample interviews selected from the many interviews with dieters that were done as part of the research for this book.

These interviews were chosen because they are typical examples of the responses of people using the starch-blocker.

Interview Number One

T.W., female, Fort Wayne, Indiana, 20 years old, housewife.

Interviewer—Are you still taking the starch-blocker?

T.W.—Only occasionally. I reached my goal weight and now I only take it when I eat a really starchy meal, or if I start to put on an extra pound or two.

Interviewer—Did you feel that the starch-blocker

was very beneficial to your successful attempt to lose weight?

T.W.—You bet! It made my diet so much more interesting and easy. I could have so many different things to eat if I took the starch-blocker, like spaghetti and corn. Some of my favorite foods were made available to me because of the starch-blocker.

Interviewer—At about what rate did you lose your weight, and how much did you lose?

T.W.—I lost it at about three pounds a week. I kept that up for about ten weeks, and knocked off around 34 pounds. My weight went from about 175 to 139. It didn't really drop tremendously fast, but the loss was real steady. I was able to stay on the weight-loss phase for a fairly long time, because my diet didn't feel that much like a diet. When I started to feel hungry, I'd sit down and have something totally tasty, like spaghetti or some tapioca pudding or something, and just take a starch-blocker with it. And I'd get hardly any calories! It was great!

Interviewer—Did the way you normally eat change much after you started using the starch-blocker?

T.W.—It did, because I started learning more about food. I learned how much starch and sugar and fat and protein were in different foods, and I found out what kinds of foods I could eat a lot of without getting fat. I eat a more balanced diet now than I used to—more varieties of foods. For a while, during the weight-loss phase of the starch-blocker program, I was eating quite a few starchy foods, to make the weight come off faster, but now I just eat a normal amount of starch.

Interviewer—Have you had a very difficult time maintaining your weight loss?

T.W.—Not at all. I've learned how to juggle starch calories so that I can occasionally eat a real heavy meal without putting on extra pounds. Even without that big meal "safety valve," though, I'm pretty satisfied almost all the time. If I take the starch-blocker, I can eat almost everything that I really want. I can eat around 2,000 calories on maintenance, as long as I block about 500 of them with the starch-blocker.

Interviewer—Do you ever feel deprived or have a strong urge to eat large amounts of sugary or fatty foods?

T.W.—You feel so much better being thin that you're really careful not to let yourself get carried away with your desires and jeopardize your new figure. So you just don't want to binge too much. Everybody's got to binge a little, but if you let yourself have that little no-no, you won't end up eating that big no-no. On other diets, where you don't get to eat as much in your maintenance phase, you're more prone to binge. On all those other diets, you get hungrier, then when you eat something to satisfy the hunger, you immediately put weight on, and that discourages you, so you eat even more. I don't care what all those diet doctors say about not getting hungry on their diets—*you get hungry!* And you eat.

Interviewer—You don't fall into the cycle of hunger-discouragement-eating on this program?

T.W.—No. This program reinforces your will power, instead of defeating it. Being able to use the starch-blocker gives you confidence in your ability to stay on top of your weight. When you use the starch-blocker, you feel like you've got an extra edge in the battle, and it just naturally makes you more able to resist temptation.

Interview Number Two

B.A., Female, Fort Wayne, Indiana, 32 years old, hospital employee.

Interviewer—Are you still using the starch-blocker regularly?

B.A.—Pretty regularly—I use about two tablets a day.

Interviewer—Are you still losing weight?

B.A.—Yes, but not as much as before, when I was taking one tablet with every meal and sometimes part of a tablet with snacks. I lost about three pounds last week, but I was losing almost a pound a day during the first three weeks.

Interviewer—Have you lost quite a bit of weight?

B.A.—Yes I have, but I still have quite a bit to go. I started at about 205, and now I'm at 175. My goal weight is 145, and I hope to reach it in about two months.

Interviewer—Have you had difficulty losing your weight?

B.A.—Not so awfully much. Every so often I see some food that really hits my fantasy, but a lot of the time it's something I can have, like a big baked potato. If I have a starch-blocker, I can eat quite a few of my food fantasies.

Interviewer—What are some of your food fantasies that you can have?

B.A.—Corn on the cob. Love it! And hash browns with onions and tomato sauce and melted cheese; and spaghetti with clam sauce. And Spanish rice, with mushrooms, stuffed into green peppers.

I'm lucky, because a lot of my favorite foods are very starchy. I've always had a real weakness for starchy foods. It used to be that they would really make me puff up, but now, if I eat them with the starch-blocker, it helps me lose weight.

Interviewer—Can you eat most of the foods the rest of your family eats?

B.A.—Most of them, yes. Like, if my family is having a steak and baked potato, I can have a big-old baked potato and just a little piece of steak. That way I don't get to feeling left out of the whole deal.

Interviewer—Had you tried many other diets before?

B.A.—I've tried them all. I usually do good for the first couple of weeks, then start to have problems. Diets tend to wear you down over a period of time; I think you don't get enough iron or vitamins or something. It just builds up. You get low and draggy, like you were undernourished. Then you feel like if you don't get something to eat, you're going to drop dead.

My resistance would sometimes get so low after a couple of weeks of dieting that I'd come down with something, like a cold, and end up in the doctor's office.

Interviewer—After you'd fall off a diet, would you tend to gain back all the weight you had lost?

B.A.—You won't believe this, but sometimes I'd gain back *double* the weight I'd lost. After I came off a diet, I'd feel like I just couldn't get enough food in me, and before I'd know it, I would be a lot heavier than before the diet. Sometimes this would happen in only about a week.

Interviewer—What other diets have you tried?

B.A.—*All* of them—you name it; I've tried it. The one I did best on was the high protein diet—you know, the all-meat one. I tried that one when I was only about 30 pounds over. But once I got to my goal weight with that one, I started eating with the family again, and, sure enough, the weight came right back on.

Interviewer—But this regaining of lost weight hasn't happened with the starch-blocker program?

B.A.—No, and I don't think it will happen, because I just don't have that old urge to get off the diet. This diet seems like normal eating to me, and I feel like keeping it up.

Interview Number Three

J.A.M., female, Bloomington, Indiana, 67 years old, retired.

Interviewer—How do you like the starch-blocker weight control program?

J.A.M.—I think it works, and I think it's great!

Interviewer—Did it make your weight loss relatively easy?

J.A.M.—To be perfectly honest, I had already lost most of the weight I needed to lose just before I heard about the starch-blocker. I was going to a clinic and was losing pretty well, then they announced the addition of the starch-blocker to their program. What has pleased me, though, is that I'm having a tremendously easy time keeping off the weight I lost.

I took off about 25 pounds on a 500-calorie per day diet, and believe me, 500 calories can be torture. You can get pretty empty on that. I would have had to stay on 500 calories, or even 1,000 or 1,200 or 1,300, I don't know if I could have kept the weight off. If past experience means anything, I can say for sure that I wouldn't have been able to have kept it off. I seem to be an easy gainer.

Interviewer—Why do you say you're an easy gainer?

J.A.M.—My doctor has told me for years that my thyroid is on the underactive side. It's not bad enough to take medicine for, but he thinks it does make me prone to be overweight.

My husband—he's retired, too—is actually less active than me, because of his arthritis, but he eats about 700 or 800 calories a day more than me without gaining weight. He's just got one of those metabolisms that can handle it.

If I eat a steady 1,200 calories a day, I can stay at about 125 to 130 pounds. But if I eat more than that, which I tend to do because I don't get filled up on 1,200 calories, I gain. I've been as high as 165. I started my current diet, the one I was on when I heard about the starch-blocker, at 155. Now my weight is 131, give or take a pound.

Interviewer—Do you feel like you will be able to keep your weight where it is?

J.A.M.—I don't see why not. I'm a fairly disciplined person, and the diet I'm eating now is no sacrifice. I actually don't care that much about food, as long as my stomach isn't growling. Meals are no big deal at our house.

Interviewer—Has using the starch-blocker changed how you eat?

J.A.M.—I can't say that it has. It mostly just keeps me from gaining when I do eat. I do tend to eat more freely now, though, when I go out. If I'm in a restaurant, I'll have the baked potato or roll or toast that they bring out. I didn't used to be able to eat those foods, which took a lot of fun out of going out to eat.

Interviewer—Do you take a starch-blocker with every meal?

J.A.M.—I used to, but I found you don't really need a whole one most of the time. As a rule, I break them in half.

Interviewer—Do you have any trouble affording the starch-blocker?

J.A.M.—I might if I took four or five a day, because we're on a fixed income. But if you use them carefully, they're just not very expensive.

Interview Number Four

D.D.S., male, Santa Clara, Oregon, 29, contractor.

Interviewer—Have you lost weight since you've started the starch-blocker program?

D.D.S.—Actually, I've gained. You probably don't want to put me in your book, because I'm not a very good success story. I can't seem to make any diet work.

Interviewer—The calorie-blocking of the starch blocker didn't help enough to make a difference in your weight?

D.D.S.—If it could block beer, it might work for

me. Starch isn't my problem. It's beer and sweets. I'm relatively compulsive about both of them—once I get started, I really don't care to stop. It's all or nothing with me. I'm one of those guys who should have his jaws wired shut.

Interviewer—How much did you gain on the starch-blocker program?

D.D.S.—Only about five pounds. The elimination of most of my starch calories helped quite a bit, but I seemed to make up for it with more desserts and more brew. I started the program at 175 and I'm at 180 now. A good weight for me would be 160, maybe 155. When I first started taking the starch-blocker, I lost about five pounds. But then I thought—aha—I can get away with murder! So I went out and bought a bunch of Sara Lee banana nut and carrot cakes because I thought they would be pretty starchy. Well, they weren't. They made my belly really puffy and gave me an even worse craving for sweets.

Interviewer—Do you consider yourself very serious about losing weight?

D.D.S.—I'm probably more serious than I act. I don't like to look fat any more than anybody else does. But you've got to keep it in perspective, right? Food—especially really well-made desserts, and good, dark beer—really give me a psychological lift. When I eat something good, I feel like I'm making up for all the aggravation from the job and from my girlfriend. I know that I'll regret it later, but that guilt somehow makes the food and beer taste even better.

Interviewer—Do you think that if you tried harder, you could decrease your caloric intake?

D.D.S.—If I ever got to where I wanted to lose weight more than I wanted to eat or drink, I imagine I could. If I was strongly motived to lose weight, I'd probably take the starch-blocker and start living on spaghetti. The product works; there's no doubt in my mind about that. I could tell it worked the first time I took it, because it made my stomach feel more full about half-way through a starchy dinner. But I'm just not a good candidate for any diet at this time in my life, because I'm not very dedicated.

Interviewer—Do you worry about the health hazards of being overweight?

D.D.S.—I'm too young to worry about that. The only thing I worry about is that women will think I look fat. I also worry a little about not holding up as well on the basketball court as I did a few years ago.

Interviewer—Have you tried other diets before?

D.D.S.—Only a diet I invented myself. I call it the On/Off Diet. I eat whatever I want one day, then absolutely nothing the next, and just alternate like that indefinitely. I can keep my weight pretty stable if I do that for a couple of months. It makes dieting easy—no thinking is involved. And this system goes well with the all-or-nothing attitude I have. The trouble with it, though, is that you only really enjoy one day out of every two. I don't need to tell you which day it is.

Interview Number Five

S.A.L., male, Indianapolis, Indiana, 56 years old, salesman.

Interviewer—How much weight have you lost on the starch-blocker program?

S.A.L.—About 32 pounds.

Interviewer—Was your weight loss difficult?

S.A.L.—On the contrary, it was easy. It was made easy because, as I lost weight, my health improved, which made me really want to keep watching what I was eating.

Interviewer—How did your health improve?

S.A.L.—Mostly, I just had more energy. That may not sound like much, but if you've ever really felt run-down and washed out for a long period of time, you can appreciate how good it is to feel like jumping out of bed in the morning again. Another thing that happened was that the arthritis in my knees seemed to feel a lot better, and my breathing improved. I had been developing sort of a wheeze, but that went away when the weight came off. I also feel better emotionally now, but that may be just because I feel better physically.

Interviewer—Had you previously related your health problems to your overweight condition?

S.A.L.—Sort of, but the weight and the health problems had come on so gradually that I didn't really put them together. After a while, you begin to take not feeling very well for granted. You start to think that everyone feels worse as they get older.

Interviewer—Had you lost weight before and felt better as a result?

S.A.L.—No, this was my first real diet. I've never felt like joining one of those weight loss groups before, because that's just not my style. I don't really believe in telling other people about my problems. Also I'm out of town too much to attend regular meetings.

I looked around at some of those popular diets—the ones on the best seller list—and anybody can tell they are phoney. Some of the clients I take out to lunch get into these things of just eating fruit or just eating meat, and they never really seem to get any thinner. Anyway, I'd feel like a nut going into a nice restaurant and ordering a bowl of oranges. If I'm with somebody and they do something like that, I feel stupid.

Interviewer—Do you just eat normal, regular food on your starch-blocker program?

S.A.L.—Sure, the same things as always, with maybe just a little bit more bread and rice and potatoes and lesser amounts of sugars and fats. I really like the starchy foods better anyway. I also tend to eat slightly more often now in Italian restaurants, which is fine with me. I hold back on the alcohol and on desserts and fatty meats such as bacon and ham. But that's no big loss. Other than that, there's nothing special about the way I eat. If I had to make a big production out of every meal, I wouldn't be on this program.

Interviewer—Was your weight loss gradual or fairly fast?

S.A.L.—Quite gradual. If I had changed my diet more, I am sure it would have been faster, but I didn't want to change my diet that much. So I just took a starch-blocker with every meal which eliminated about twenty percent of my calories.

Interviewer—You were in no hurry to lose the weight?

S.A.L.—No. And now I'm in no hurry to gain it back!

NOTE

Since the introduction of my original SLPC Starch-Blocker* product many imitators have appeared in the market. Dieters should be aware that product quality differences exist.

The unique technology and rigid processing method that I have developed during twelve years of research meets the highest standard that assures consistent product quality and activity. It is important that the product contain sufficient activity to inhibit the digestion of the stated quantity of starch. Extensive comparative analyses have been done by independent laboratories of products currently available in the market. There are great differences in these products, even to the extent that some products are nothing more than ground beans. Such products may be harmful since toxins have not been removed. For more information, send a self-addressed and stamped envelope to the publisher. Symbion Press, P.O. Box 2896, Batesville, AR 72501.

J. John Marshall, Ph.D.

*Starch-Blocker is a Trademark of Dynavest

The following Starch-Blocker products are recommended:

CARBO-LITE
CALOREX
ALPHA-PLEX
REDU-CAL
SERIOLAC